MEDICAL TERMINOLOGY
BY THE
MNEMONIC STORY SYSTEM

MEDICAL TERMINOLOGY

BY THE

MNEMONIC STORY SYSTEM

WILLIAM J RUSSELL

To order additional copies of this book, contact:
Xlibris Corporation
1-888-795-4274
www.Xlibris.com
Orders@Xlibris.com
34605

CONTENTS

INTRODUCTION TO THE MNEMONIC STORY SYSTEM OF LEARNING MEDICAL TERMINOLOGY

This introduction is for those taking the self-learning course using the book only. The mnemonic story learning system allows a student to study at his or her own leisure. Taking time as needed. However, in order to fully understand this system, it is best to read all material. Therefore, you should read both introductions. This will give you an idea how the course is taught.

Start by reading chapter one. This chapter gives a brief introduction into how words are put together, and gives clue to some of the ways for pronunciation, spelling, and rules for plurals. A medical word can be complex. It is like a chemical compound. Elements make up words. Words then, become compounds (by analogy). For instance, take the compound sodium chloride. It is made up of two elements, sodium Na and chlorine Cl. Sodium is a caustic metal that is harmful to the touch, and chlorine is a gas that is deadly poisonous. However, when combined they form sodium chloride, common table salt, but a necessary ingredient for life. Medical words are much the same. Often when the elements are separate, they mean one thing, when put together, something quite different.

The process of learning in this book is in three parts. First, you must commit to memory the mnemonic device. Second, you must familiarize yourself with the association-image, a kind of short story paragraph. Third, you must now be able to identify the mnemonic device in a story that refers to a medical word element. It sounds horrific. It is not. Starting with chapter four, and thereafter, there will be a short story following each 3 chapters. These stories are part of your testing. After studying the chapters, test yourself with the stories. Answers appear in the appendix section. But, do not look at them until you have tried all the paragraphs in each story.

You are wondering if that is all that there is to it. Right! Well, not quite. In order for you to have a working knowledge of the elements, you must make up flash cards. It is quite a process. On one side is the medical element. On the reverse side, is the meaning and the mnemonic device? If you want to get very fancy, makes up a second group of cards with the association-image on one side and the meaning, or medical element, on the other side. The idea is to give your memory an anchor, somewhere in your mind to help you find the word of reference.

angi-o-	**VESSEL, USUALLY BLOOD** Angie—When angie does her daily exercise the blood vessels in her legs stand out like mini road maps.
FRONT	**BACK**

INTRODUCTION TO
THE MNEMONIC STORY SYSTEM
OF LEARNING FOR CLASSROOM

What is a mnemonic system of learning, anyway? Well, it is a system of learning that uses sound-alike words as devices to stimulate memory recall. The mnemonic device, along with an association/image, assists the learner with remembering. In this text there are 300 word elements. These elements, when learned, will allow the learner to have access to well over eight thousand-word compounds. In addition, along with the mnemonic device will be given stories written using the association/image descriptions. These stories, also used as testing motifs, will give the learner practice in element recognition, as well as element meaning, to a growing number of medical terms.

Classroom lectures/discussion will review the material one 30-element lesson at a time. 300 elements will be reviewed. There will be three 100-element tests and one 90-element (plus 10 story questions making 100 in all) final. The first 100-element test begins with the element ab- and ends with the element gingiv-; the second 100-element test begins with the element glom- and ends with the element -penia; the last 100-element test begins with the element peps- and ends with the element vulse-. The final exam will have 90 elements taken at random from the ten lessons plus ten story questions. This makes for 100 questions in all. The primary difference between the final exam and the three tests is that the final does not have any bonus questions. What you see is what you get. On the first three 100-word element tests there will also be story questions. These questions will be in addition to the 100-word elements and be counted as bonus questions. Bonus questions allow for you to pick up either additional points or to assist you with points lost on the 100-word element test due to incorrect answers. If you score 100% on the test and score one to ten bonus points, the bonus points can be carried forward to the next test. Another way to gain extra points is to create three stories yourself during the first 12 weeks of the course. This can be done by following the example given in the book. Remember, in order to receive the extra points you must follow the format suggested in the book. During the first 12 weeks you can acquire only 30 points by creating three stories. Each story must have no more than 10 elements used in not more than three lessons. Read the examples given in this text: Practical Exercise in the Story Test and Practice Makes Perfect. If you have any questions, please ask the instructor during a break time.

To assist with the learning process and to put some of the words into a living model, there will be lectures within the following disciplines: Neuropsychiatry, Orthopaedics, Cardiology, Pharmacology, and special procedures if time permits. There is also time allowed for student choice subjects, if time allows, and the instructor has the knowledge! Spelling Bees can be scheduled and spelling quizzes are scheduled as shown in the syllabus.

Regarding class discipline and test taking to include makeups: It is expected that students who attend this class will come to learn, and not to visit with their friends. To this end students who talk while the class is in progress shall do so at the risk of being asked to leave the classroom. After three such instances a failing grade shall be given. This excludes asking and answering questions consonant with class subjects. All homework is due on the date specified/assigned. Late work is subject to accrue a loss of percentage of the assigned grade (<100%). Tests are taken on the assigned dates unless the instructor makes exceptions. Tests (to include spelling quizzes on audio tapes) shall be left in the Learning Center for those unable to be present on the test date. The tests left at the Learning Center will be there on the night of the test and will be picked up at the next class date or one week which ever is later. Three missed consecutive classes may be cause for failure of the course or for a student to be dropped by the instructor.

Please read the assignments and try the method. I have often heard the saying, "But I don't like this method." While it is certainly true that not everyone finds this system enjoyable, it is also true that if one tries, one will learn in spite of oneself. So try and try once more. The material given is time tested.

The written assignment is worth two grade points. Yes, *two* grade points. It is not a graded assignment. You will get the points just by doing the assignment. Please do so. It is also very important that you read this entire book. Everything that you will need to know is here. It is especially important that you attend class. While it is possible to pass this course by studying the book only, with the additional information given in class you will do much better. The average grade when using the book is 72 percent, while the average for those who attend class is 88 percent. If you fail, a re-test can be given. However, both scores, the failed and the re-test, will be averaged together. That will then be your grade for that test. Using the Learning Center is only for those who are unable to attend class for an honest reason. Please do not come to class, tell me that you have not studied, and want to take the test later. That is unfair for those who have prepared for the test. You will certainly know when each test is to be given and that means having time to prepare for the test. There are no secrets in this class. All is given.

Regarding the ten lessons, third hour apperception exercises. You will notice on page six that you get ten points for attending these hours. However, if you miss any of these hours, or leave early, you will not get the point for the third hour. These hours can be made up by writing 15 sentences, each with a different medical word taken from the exercise page. However, these sentences must have the medical word used in the correct context. Reference: F. *Assignments That Demonstrate Critical Thinking*, 2. Given a medical term use the term/word in a written or spoken sentence demonstrating an understanding of the meaning of the term/word by creating a new sentence using the term/word.

Example: 1. Cardiology: My friend had a heart condition and therefore his doctor sent him to the *cardiology* clinic.

As you can see, first the word is identified, then it is defined by correct use in a sentence. If you have questions about this makeup assignment, please ask the instructor.

Please read next the syllabus.

SYLLABUS (for classroom instruction)

SUBJECT AREA AND COURSE NUMBER (To be designated)

COURSE TITLE: Medical Terminology

CATALOG DESCRIPTION:

To furnish an understanding of the need and reason for the technical language of medicine. To demonstrate how terms come into being and how they are used and formed. To build a background vocabulary in medical terminology and demonstrate a complete word building system using mnemonic (memory) devices or phrases that make it easy for the user to understand and remember a growing medical terminology.

CLASS SCHEDULE DESCRIPTION:

Give yourself the power of understanding and using medical terminology. When your doctor says, "The patient must refrain from heterosexual interdigitation." You can say, "Is that so the dactylitis won't become dactylosymphysis?" Enroll in Medical Terminology today!

STUDENT OUTCOMES/OBJECTIVES:

The student will learn ways to understand, interpret, transcribe (limited), speak, and write complex medical terms during the course, and:

1. Given a medical term, divide the term into suffix, prefix and stem; saying out loud with correct pronunciation; or, distinguish the meaning by writing a meaning synonym on a test or to do so by stating the meaning out loud in class.
2. Given a medical term use the term/word in a written or spoken sentence demonstrating an understanding of the term/word.

COURSE CONTENT AND SCOPE:

A.   CHAPTERS

1. Ten lessons each with 30 word elements creating an access to over 8,000 medical words.
2. Each lesson of 30 word elements (suffixes, prefixes and stems) given with their meanings.
3. During the course, all students will be given the opportunity to pronounce and define compound words made from the word elements found in one or more lessons. Elements are introduced in alphabetical order. This will allow for an increasing number of made-up words in each lesson, giving the student more words to practice with for each succeeding lesson.

B.   LECTURE INFORMATION WITH TOPICS: (For full Semester Courses)

1. Orthopaedics
2. Neuropsychiatry
3. General Surgical/Anatomical Descriptions
4. Cardiology
5. Example of transcription format in psychiatry (Intake Format)

C.   READING ASSIGNMENTS:

Students will be required to read/study assigned chapters in textbook and/or handouts.

Assigned library reading may be used to substitute for lost time.

D.   WRITING ASSIGNMENTS:

In 500 words, but not less than 350 words, write an article that relates to the use of medical terminology in student's life. This should be written in essay format. For more information on this writing assignment please read Writing Assignment. Substantial writing assignments in this course are inappropriate because the Mnemonic System deals with writing as its primary concern, as will be evidenced by many assignments.

E.   OUT OF CLASSROOM ASSIGNMENTS/STUDY:

Two (2) hours study/work outside of class for each hour in class is advised. Three (3) tests of 100-word elements and one (1) final of a mixture of word elements and phrases (association/images) given in class. One (1) outside paper of 500 words, no less than 350. Extra credit assignments consisting of creating stories using the format suggested in Practice Makes Perfect and Practical Exercise in Story Test.

F.   ASSIGNMENTS THAT DEMONSTRATE CRITICAL THINKING:

Students will demonstrate the ability to think critically by performing the following tasks:

1. Given a compound medical word, divide into suffix, prefix and stem; say the meaning aloud or write a meaning synonym on a test; or do so in class, by stating the meaning aloud after correct pronunciation of the compound medical word.
2. Given a medical term, use the term/word in a written or spoken sentence demonstrating an understanding of the meaning of the term/word by creating a new sentence using the term/word.
3. On a test, given the medical element/term define the element in lay terms. Example: For cardi give the response heart.
4. Identify word elements when introduced in a written paragraph of association/ images with mnemonic device taken from lessons, in a story format, by defining the element.

Example: The card was the ace of hearts. Mnemonic device is card. The medical term is cardi. Meaning is heart. On a story test, you would be looking for the medical element. Turn to the story in the Practical Exercise in the Story Test (Beauty and the Ace). Read the story and see if you can figure out the medical word elements being referred to in the story. There are eight.

G.   METHOD OF INSTRUCTION:

Lecture with discussion time for students to reply to questions regarding meaning. Time in the classroom for the student to demonstrate correct enunciation and pronunciation by using spelling bees and other out-loud tasks to assist with the evaluation of the student's growing vocabulary of medical words. Periodic written examinations as shown. Specific discipline-related terminology during lectures. Visual flash cards used during presentation of 30-element lessons with ad lib data given as questions arise.

H.   METHODS OF EVALUATION:

Three (3) 100-element tests = 40% of grade; one (1) final = 40% of grade; four (4) spelling quizzes = 8% of grade; classroom verbal exercises = 10%, 1% for each lesson; and, one (1) paper = 2% of grade. Grades: D = 60-69%; C = 70-79%; B = 80-89%; and, A = 90-100%. 30 points can be earned by doing extra story tests. These points can then be used to bring

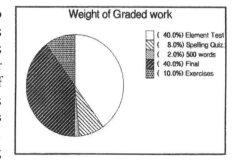

Weight of Graded work

(40.0%) Element Test
(8.0%) Spelling Quiz
(2.0%) 500 words
(40.0%) Final
(10.0%) Exercises

up low scores on element tests, and the final exam only. For distant learning classes, 50% for 3 tests, and 50% for final.

I.   TEXT: Medical Terminology by the Mnemonic Story System, W. J. Russell, LVN, present Edition.

J.   REPEATABLE FOR CREDIT: YES (X)

This course teaches a basic vocabulary in medical terminology. It is possible that there will be students that may want to repeat this course as a refresher only. At this time the course being presented is by a text the Medical Terminology by the *Mnemonic Story System.*

MEDICAL TERMINOLOGY
WEEKLY SCHEDULE
(For full semester schedule)

1. Date_____
   Introduction (*Zero Week*)
   Assignment: read Introduction, Syllabus, Writing Assignment;
   Study Chapter One before class.
   Lecture _____

2. Date_____
   First lesson of 30 terms (1) in class
   Quiz on reading assignment
   Home study lesson (2)

3. Date_____
   30 terms lesson (2) in class
   Answer questions
   Home study lesson (3)

4. Date_____
   30 terms lesson (3) in class
   Spelling quiz (1E) Lesson 2
   Home study lesson (4)

5. Date_____
   30 terms lesson (4) in class
   Med-term abbreviations
   Home work assignment: 500 words
   Home study lesson (5)

6. Date_____
   First 100 Element Test (ab- to gingiv-) After lecture
   Lecture: Schizophrenia (I or II)
   Turn in home work assignment 500 words
   Review

7. Date_____
   30 terms lesson (5) in class
   Elective Lecture _____
   Home study lesson (6)

8. Date_____   30 terms lesson (6) in class
                         Spelling quiz (2W) Lesson 4_____
                         Home study lesson (7)

9. Date_____   30 terms lesson (7) in class
                         Elective lecture _____
                         Home study lesson (8)

10. Date_____   *Second 100 Element test (glom- to -penia)*
                         Lecture: Orthopaedics terms/specialty
                         Home study lesson (8)

11. Date_____   30 terms lesson (8) in class
                         Spelling quiz (3E) Lesson 6_____
                         Lecture: Communication Theory
                         Home study lesson (9)

12. Date_____   30 terms lesson (9) in class
                         Elective lecture _____
                         Home study lesson (10)

13. Date_____   30 terms lesson (10) in class
                         Lecture: Cardiology

14. Date_____   *Third 100 Element test (peps- to vulse-)*
                         Lecture: Pharmacology

15. Date_____   Spelling quiz (4W) Lesson 8_____
                         Lecture/Discussion Dental
                         Read section in text before this lecture and
                         bring in questions on paper (hand in after class)

16. Date_____   Preparation for final exam
                         Review _____

17. Date_____   Final Examination _____

18. Date_____   Final Examination (When there are 18 days)

WRITING ASSIGNMENT
(For Classroom Instruction)

In 500 words, or no less than 350, write an essay that relates to the use of medical terminology in your life. The essay should give clue to your reason for taking medical terminology and how this course will fit in with your future. Identify your motivation. Clarify your goal. Tell me what it is that you plan to achieve.

An essay is a brief documentation or short literary composition on a single subject, usually presenting the personal view of the author; in some cases, an assigned topic by a teacher, but nevertheless, even though an assignment, still presenting the personal view of the author. Often the topic given by the teacher allows for the author's view in one of several ways.

As I have stated in the first paragraph, I have chosen the way you will respond by asking several questions. Perhaps these questions will assist you with clarification of your goal choice. At the very least, this assignment should make you think. My motivation for having you write this essay is to get to know each of you a little better. One of the fundamental essentials for the acquisition of knowledge is the ability to write; therefore, the reason and the motivation behind your writing something that I can read. The essay may be two (2) grade points, but it can assist me in the evaluation process. Often students have difficulty with this style of learning. Sometimes reviewing your writing may give me a clue to the reason why. After all, the primary reason we are here at all is to learn. Learning about how we process knowledge may help us in our future endeavors.

I must insist that you do this assignment. If you have a doubt in your mind, now is the time to remove it. Do not hesitate to ask questions. If you choose not to do this assignment, it is not just two grade points that you will lose, you may also not find out the reason that you are having difficulty with this subject. Medical terminology is a language by itself. If you are going to be working in the profession, you will need to speak the language.

CHAPTER ONE

A Beginning in Word Recognition For Medical Terminology

"SOUNDS LIKE" PRONUNCIATION

A new medical term is much easier to comprehend and remember when you can pronounce it properly. To assist with this process, each new term in this book will be identified (in parentheses) by a phonetic spelling.

A WORD OF CAUTION

There are different ways to pronounce many medical terms. The ones shown in this book are ones found most commonly. Your instructor may prefer a different pronunciation. This will not necessarily mean that the ones shown are wrong. Often both pronunciations are correct, and it is simply a matter of personal preference or a reflection of an individual's background and education.

SPELLING IS ALWAYS IMPORTANT

Accuracy in spelling medical terms is very important!

Changing as little as one letter can create a completely different word. Both sound-alike and close spelling can cause errors in transcription as shown by the following words.

Synostosis = Union between adjacent bones of a single bone.
Sinistrosis = Shell shock (old term from 2nd world war)

Coleocystitis = Inflammation of the bladder and vagina.
Cholecystitis = Inflammation of the gall bladder.

Hysteroid = Resembling hysteria.
Histoid = Like a tissue of the body.

Hysterolysis = Loosening of the uterus from its attachments or adhesions.
Histolysis = Breaking down of tissue.

Formication = Sensation of ants creeping upon the skin; a form of paresthesia.
Fornication = Sexual intercourse between unmarried partners.

MEDICAL DICTIONARY USE

In the study of medical terminology, you will learn to unravel the meanings of compound words by breaking them down into their elements. However, some terms may defy this process. Even words that seem obvious based on their elements may have more than one meaning. For example, look up the term *cardiectomy* (kar-dee-ECK-toh-me).

- Based on the word elements, cardiectomy sounds like it means removal of the heart. (the combining form cardio- means heart and the suffix -ectomy means removal of all of all or part).

  However, when you use a medical dictionary the meaning is: (cardiectomy) Excision of the cardiac end of the stomach. It is possible that today one might use this term to Describe what is done during a heart transplant; as the part of the operation that precedes the actual surgical attachment of the heart into another person.

  Another example is the term *lithotomy* (lih-THOT-oh-me).

- Based on the word parts, lithotomy means a surgical incision for the removal of a stone. (The combining form lith/0 means stone and the suffix -otomy means a surgical incision.
- Lithotomy is also the name of an examination position in which the patient is lying on the Back with the feet and legs raised and supported in stirrups.

If You Know How To Spell the Word

- If you are sure of the first three letters you can usually find the word. However, if you are Not, the following chart may help you with the spelling of words by how they sound.

TABLE ONE

Sounds Like	It May Begin With	Example	Phonetics
F Sound	F PH	Flatus Phlegm	FLAY-tus FLEM
J Sound	G J	Gingivitis Jaundice	Jin-jih-VYE-tis JAWN-dis
K Sound	C CH K QU	Crepitus Cholera Kyphosis Quadriplegia	KREP-ih-tus KOL-er-ah Kye-FOH-sis Kwad-rih-plee-jee-ah
S Sound	C PS S	Cytology Psychology Serology	Sigh-TOL-oh-jee Sigh-KOL-oh-jee She-ROL-oh-jee
Z Sound	X Z	Xeroderma Zygote	Zee-roh-DER-mah ZYE-goht

In the space provided below write other examples you have found:

_____

_____

_____

_____

_____

_____

_____

_____

_____

Singular and Plural Endings

- Many medical terms have Greek and Latin origins. Because of these different origins there are unusual rules for changing a singular word into a plural form. Also, English endings have been adopted for some commonly used terms. Table Two will assist your understanding of this process.

TABLE TWO

On The Matter of Pluralizing

1. if the term ends in A, the plural is formed by adding an E	bursa	Bursae
2. if the term ends in EX or IX, the plural is formed by changing the EX or IX to ICES	Appendix	Appendices
3. if the term ends in IS, the plural is formed by changing the IS to ES	diagnosis metastasis	diagnoses metastases
4. if the term ends in IT IS, the plural is formed by dropping the S and adding DES	arthritis meningitis	arthritides meningitides
5. if the term ends in NX, the plural is formed by changing the X to G and adding ES	phalanx	phalanges
6. if the term ends in ON, the plural is formed by dropping the ON and adding A	criterion	criteria
7. if the term ends in UM, the plural is formed by changing the UM to A	diverticulum datum	diverticula data
8. if the term ends in US, the plural is formed by changing the US to I	alveolus malleolus	alveoli malleoli

Figure One

A phalanx is one finger or toe bone. Two or more of these bones are called phalanges.

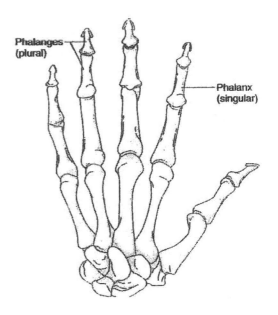

WORD ELEMENTS

Many medical terms are made from more than one element. Much like chemical compounds, medical terms are made from elements joined together to produce a new compound word. Learning medical terminology is accomplished faster once you know the many parts, or the elements used to build words. The types of parts are:

- Prefixes that usually, but not always, indicate location, time, number, or status.
- Combining forms that usually, but not always, indicate the involved body part.
- Suffixes that usually, but not always, indicate the procedure, condition, disorder, or disease.

In this book there are many, over 300, word elements. These elements will give you access to as many as 8,000 words. Starting in chapter two you will be given these elements in alphabetical order. Figure two below will show you in blocking format how words can be thought to be pieced together.

Figure Two

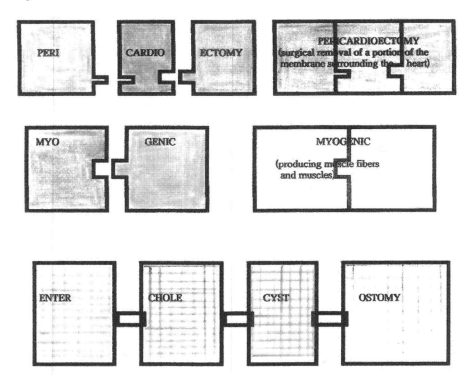

Entercholecystostomy (enter-koh-lee-sist-ahs-toh-me) surgical creation of an artificial passage between the intestine and gallbladder.

PREFIXES

A prefix is added to the beginning of a word to change the meaning of the term. As said before, prefixes usually, but not always, indicate location, time, or number. See table three.

TABLE THREE

CONTRASTING AND CONFUSING PREFIXES

Without a prefix the root **febril** *(Feb-ril)* Means having fever	**A**—means away from, negative, and without. **Afebrile** *(ay-Feb-ril)* means without fever.
AB—means away from. **Abnormal** means not Normal or away from normal.	**AD**—means toward or in the direction of. **Addiction** means drawn toward strong dependence on a drug or substance.
DYS—means difficult, painful or bad. **Dysfunctional** means an organ or body part that is not working properly.	**EU**—means well, easy, or good. **Eupnea** *(youp-NEE-ah)* means easy or normal Breathing. (the suffix—PNEA means breathing)
HYPER—means over, above, or increased. **Hypertension** *(high-per-TEN-shun)* higher than normal blood pressure.	**HYPO**—means below, under, or decreased. **Hypotension** *(high-poh-TEN-shun)* lower than normal blood pressure.
INTER—means between or among. **Interstit-Ial** (in-ter-STISH-al) means within the parts of body tissue.	**INTRA**—means within. **Intramuscular** (in-trah-MUS-kyou-lar) means within the muscle.
POLY—means many. **Polyuria** *(pol-ee-YOU-ree-ah)* means excessive urination. **URIA**—means urination.	**OLIG/O**—a combining form, means few, scant, or little **Oliguria** *(ol-ih-GOO-ree-ah)* means scanty or infrequent urination.
SUB—means under, less, or below. **Subcostal** *(sub-kos-tal)*—means below a rib or ribs. (The combining form **COST/O** means rib or ribs.	**SUPER**—and **SUPRA**—both mean above, excessive, or beyond. **Supracostal** *(sue-prah-KOS-tal)* means obove or outside the ribs.

COMBINING FORMS

Combining forms, sometimes called the body or root, usually, but not always, describe the part of the body part that is involved. See tables four and five.

Combining forms are used with prefixes, other combining forms, and suffixes to create new words. See below.

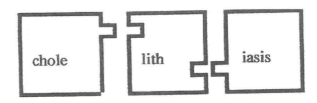

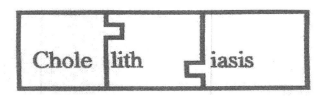

In the foregoing example the term is cholelithiasis. It is made up of the:

- Prefix chole- meaning bile.
- Combining form lith meaning stone.
- Suffix -iasis meaning condition.

Cholelithiasis (kol-lee-lih-THIGH-ah-sis) is the presence of gallstones in the gallbladder or bile ducts (The suffix -lithiasis means the presence of stones.)

Table Four

COMMONLY USED COMBINING FORMS INDICATING COLOR	
CYAN/O means blue	Cyanosis (sigh-ah-NO-sis) is bluish discoloration of the skin caused by a lack of adequate oxygen.
ERYTH/O means red	Erythrocytes (eh-RITH-roh-sites) are mature red blood cells.
LEUK/O means white	Leukocytes (LOO-koh-sites) are white blood cells.
MELAN/O means black	Melanosis (mel-ah-NO-sis) is any condition of unusual deposits of black pigment in different parts of the body.
POLI/O means gray	Poliomyelitis (poh-lee-oh-my-eh-LYE-tis) is a viral infection of the gray matter of the spinal cord that may result in paralysis.

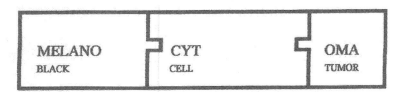

Melanocytoma (mel-ah-no-site-oh-ma) A rare pigmented benign tumor of the optic disk.

The Combining Vowel

A combining vowel may be used to modify the spelling so that the new word is easier to pronounce. The basic rules determine when the combining vowel is, or is not, used.

The combining vowel *is not used* when the suffix begins with a vowel. For example, when the combining form NEUR/O is joined with the suffix -ALGIA, the resulting term is neuralgia. Because the suffix -ALGIA begins with a vowel, the combining "o" is not used.

Neuralgia (new-RAL-jee-ah) is pain in a nerve or nerves.

The combining form *is used* when the suffix begins with a consonant. An example, when NEUR/O is joined with -PLASTY, they form neuroplasty. Because the suffix -PLASTY begins with a consonant, the combining "o" is used.

Neuroplasty (NEW-row-plas-tee) is the surgical repair of a nerve. (The combining form NEUR/O means nerve. The suffix -PLASTY means surgical repair.)

SUFFIXES

A suffix is added to the end of a combining form. Suffixes usually, but not always, indicate the procedure, condition, disorder, or disease. For example, the combining form PHARYNG/O means throat. The suffix -ITIS means inflammation and indicates a condition. Pharyngitis is an inflammation of the throat.

Several suffixes all mean "pertaining to or relating to." These suffixes, table five, usually convert a combining form into a root word.

TABLE FIVE

SUFFIX	MEANING
-AC	Cardiac arrest (KAR-dee-ack) means pertaining to the sudden stopping of the heart. (The combining form CARDI/O means heart.)
-AL	Renal failure (REE-nal) means pertaining to the failure of the kidneys. (The combining form REN/O means kidney.)
-EAL	Esophageal (eh-sof-ah-JEE-al) means pertaining to the esophagus. (The combining form ESOPHAG/O means esophagus.)
-IC	Gastric (GAS-trick) means pertaining to the stomach. (The combining form GASTR/O means stomach.)
-OUS	Cutaneous (kyou-TAY-nee-us) means pertaining to the skin. (The combining form CUTANE/O means skin.)
-TIC	Nephrotic (neh-FROT-ick) means pertaining to the kidneys. (The combining form NEPHR/O means kidney.)

Suffixes Related to Procedures

TABLE SIX

SUFFIX	MEANING
-CENTESIS	Surgical puncture to remove fluid.
-ECTOMY	Surgical removal of all or part.
-GRAPHY	Recording of a picture or making a record.
-GRAM or -GRAPH	Both to describe the resulting record or picture.
-OLOGY	Means the study of.
-OSTOMY	To surgically create an opening, a stoma, mouth.
-OTOMY	Means cutting into or a surgical incision.
-PLASTY	Means surgical repair.
-SCOPY	Means to see or a visual examination.

LOOK-ALIKE SOUND-ALIKE TERMSAND WORD PARTS

One confusing part of learning medical terminology is dealing with words that sound and look-alike. The following illustration will highlight some of the most common ones. You will certainly see many of these as you continue on your way to learning medical terminology.

Arteri/o, Ather/o, and Arthr/o	The combining form Arteri/o means artery. The combining form Ather/o means plaque or fatty substance. The combining form Arthr/o means joint.
ileum and ilium	The ileum (ILL-ee-um) is part of the small intestine (The combining form ILE/O means ileum.) (Remember, ileum with an e refers to ENTER/O that means small intestine.) The ilium (ILL-ee-um) is part of the hipbone. (The combining form ILI/O means ilium.) (Remember, ilium with an i refers to the hipbone.)
Laceration and lesion	A laceration (lass-er-AY-shun) is a torn, ragged wound. A lesion (LEE-zhun) is a pathological change of tissue due to disease or injury.
Mucous and Mucus	Mucous (MYOU-kus) describes the mucous membranes that line the body cavities. Mucus (MYOU-kus) is the substance secreted by the mucous membranes.
Myc/o, Myel/o, and My/o	The combining form MYC/O means fungus. The combining form MYEL/O means both bone marrow and spinal cord. The combining form MY/O means muscle.
Palpation and Palpitation	Palpation (pal-PAY-shun) is an examination technique in which the examiner's hands are used to feel the texture, size, consistency, and location of certain body parts/organs. Palpitation (pal-pih-TAY-shun) is a pounding or racing heart.

Prostate and Prostrate	Prostate (PROS-tayt) means a gland surrounding the neck of the bladder and urethra in the male. Prostrate (PROS-trayt) means to collapse or to be overcome with exhaustion.
Pyel/o and Py/o	The combining form PYEL/O means renal pelvis. The combining form PY/O means pus.
Supination and Suppuration	Supination (soo-pih-NAY-shun) is the act of rotating the arm so the palm of the hand is forward or upward. Suppuration (sup-you-RAY-shun) is the formation or the discharge of a pus exudate.
Suturing and Ligation	Suturing is the act of closing a wound by stitching. Ligation is the act of binding or tying off blood vessels or ducts.
Trocar and Trochanter	A trocar (TROH-kar) is a sharp, pointed surgical instrument. A trochanter (tro-KAN-ter) is one of the two large bony projections on the upper end of the femur just below the femoral neck.
Viral and Virile	Viral (VYE-ral) means pertaining to a virus. Virile (VIR-ill) means having masculine traits.

CHAPTER TWO

MNEMONICS

ELEMENT	MNEMONIC DEVICE	ASSOCIATION-IMAGE	MEANING
ab- (ab)	able	Although an *able* combat veteran Joe could not get far enough *away from* spiders. It was a real phobia.	*away from, not*

This prefix takes the form a- before m, p, and v, and abs- before c and t.

	Examples:	abnormal—away from normal; departing from normal abneural—passing away from a nerve (usually to a muscle) avulsion—"a pulling away from," as in an avulsion fracture. abscond—to run away from, esp. to freedom.	
acoust(i)- (a-coost-ee)	A costly	I *hear* that the movie with the new *sound* is a costly production.	*hearing, sound*

Because of the familiarity of acousti- in words, this form has been chosen to present the root in this form. However, the basic root meaning sound is acous- or acus-.

	Example:	-acusis—used to denote a condition of hearing (also *-acusia*)	
acro- (ak-row)	acronym	Imagine the acronym SCUBA with extremities swimming under water. *or peak.*	*extremities; tip; end a top*

Note that whatever the reference, "extremity" or acro- always includes the farthest ends and all parts leading to the farthest ends.

aden- (a-den)	laden	Certain parts of our body are laden with glands that function to fulfill a specific function.	*gland (e.g. urine)*

ELEMENT	MNEMONIC DEVICE	ASSOCIATION-IMAGE	MEANING

| | Examples: | adenic—pertaining to a gland or the glands. adenopathy—any disease of a gland. adenosis—any condition of a gland. | |

| adnexa- (ad-neks-ah) | add next | You may add next the following: two ties connected with a red bow. | *ties, connections appendages or adjacent parts* |

This word is a combination of the prefix ad- meaning "to" plus the root nex- meaning "join." Literally, the word means "joined to" and is applied chiefly to refer to the ocular adnexa, the appendages to the eye such as the lacrimal apparatus, and the uterine adnexa, the appendages or adjacent parts of the womb such as the ovaries, the uterine tubes and ligaments.

| | Examples: | adnexopexy (adnex/o/pexy)—the operation of fixing the uterine adnexa to the abdominal wall adnexitis (adnex/itis)—inflammation of the uterine adnexa | |

| aer- (ay-er) | are | He said, "You are nothing but a windbag, Sir, full of hot air." | *air* |

| | Examples: | Aerial—pertaining to air aeropathy (aer/o/pathy)—"bends" aerosis (aer/o/sis)—production of gas in the tissues or organs | |

| -algia (al-jee-ah) | Al, gee | Oh Al, gee, I wish you no pain, but you're on my foot. | *pain, painful condition* |

The element-algia may be further separated into two parts: Literally (-ia) "condition of" and (alg-) "pain,"—*algia* is the most frequent form expressing pain. However, *alg-* is a root meaning "pain" and can appear in other forms such as algesi-, algo-, algeo- algio-.

| | Examples: | algospasm (alg/o/spasm)—painful, involuntary contraction; painful cramp algiomuscular (algi/o/muscular)—causing painful muscular movements myalgia (my/algia)—pain in muscle | |

ELEMENT	MNEMONIC DEVICE	ASSOCIATION-IMAGE	MEANING
alveol- (al-vee-ol)	Al & Viola	Al & Viola are having a sock-it to me contest to see who can hit the other in the solar plexus cavity.	*cavity, socket small cavity, pit or hollow*

This root is used most frequently to refer to the cavities or sockets of either jaw in which the roots of the teeth are embedded.

| | Examples: | alveolus (alveol/us)—(plural alveoli) name used to designate a small saclike pit or cavity; dental alveoli—the tooth sockets in the upper and lower jaw bones
alveolar (alveol/ar)—pertaining to an alveolus | |

| ambi- ambo- (am-bee-oh) | Bambi | Bambi seemed trapped. There was a bamboo fence on both sides, but he was able to jump the smallest one to safety. | *both, on both sides around* |

You may know that ambi/dextrous means equal ease in using both hands. Compare with the concept extrovert and introvert. What would an ambivert be?

| | Examples: | ambi/sexual—pertaining to or affecting both sexes
ambi/ent—surrounding, on both or all sides | |

| ameb- (ah-me'bah) | ameba | When looking through a microscope you can see the one-cell'ed ameba change shape as it moves. | *change* |

| | Examples: | ameba, amoeba (ameb/a, amoeb/a)—a one-celled animal which moves by constantly changing its shape
amebic (ameb/ic)—pertaining to, or of the nature of, an ameba
amebiasis (ameb/ia/sis)—infestation with amebas, especially intestine | |

| amphi- ampho- (am'fe) | Am free | Some say I am free because I can move around on both sides of my internal world of mind; left and right, as if in two ways of thinking. | *both, in two ways, roundabout, around* |

ELEMENT	MNEMONIC DEVICE	ASSOCIATION-IMAGE	MEANING

An amphi/theater is an oval U-shaped structure surrounded by rows of seats. An amphi/bi/an can live in two environments.

	Examples:	amphi/cran/ia—pain on both sides of the head (Taber's) amph/o/dipl/op/ia—double vision in both eyes	
an-, a- (an)	an a	John brought home a report card without an A, not one A. Was he lacking in some way?	*without, not/ lacking; weakness; deficiency*
	Note:	The form of the prefix is an- before vowels (a, e, i, o, u and usually h); the form is a- before the consonants.	
	Examples:	anemia (an/em/ia)—"lack of blood"; lack of red cells in blood anesthesia (an/esthesia)—"lack of feeling"; unconsciousness avitaminosis (a/vitamin/osis)—"lack of vitamins"; vitamin deficiency atrophy (a/trophy)—"lacking development, growth"; a wasting away	
angi- (an'je)	Angie	When Angie does her daily exercise the blood vessels in her legs stand out like mini road maps.	*vessel, usually blood*
	Note:	While the principal reference is to blood vessels, angi- can also designate tubes, ducts, or canals which convey the fluids of the body.	
	Examples:	angiitis (angi/itis)—inflammation of a vessel, usually blood angiomegaly (angi/o/megal/y)—enlargement of the vessels angiosis (angi/osis)—any condition of the vessels	
ante- (an'tee)	anteup	In the card game of poker you usually anteup with your bet before the cards are dealt.	*before, before in time; or in space*
	Note:	This prefix appears in a much-used form of anter/o- which is restricted to the meaning "before in space" or "forward" usually meaning *direction*.	

ELEMENT	MNEMONIC DEVICE	ASSOCIATION-IMAGE	MEANING
	Examples:	antepartum (ante/part/um)—occurring before birth anterior (anter/ior)—situated more toward the front, belly surface anteroposterior (anter/o/poster/ior)—from front to back as in AP & Lat film	
anti- (an'tie)	auntie	I hear that your Auntie Elsie is against abortion.	*against, opposing, (acting against)*
	Examples:	antigen (anti/gen)—a substance that, when introduced into the body, stimulates the "production of" an "opposing" substance called an anti/body antalgesic (ant-al-je'-sik)—pain-relieving agent antacid (ant/acid)—a substance that counteracts acidity	
antr- (an'ter)	enter	Said the spider to the fly, "Enter my chamber and we shall see what cavity have thee!"	*cavity or chamber*
	Examples:	antrum (antr/um)—a sinus; a cavity or chamber, especially bone antrodynia (antr/o/dyn/ia)—pain in an antrum	
arthr- (ar"thro)	Arthur	King Arthur exclaimed, "It's water on my knee; I doubt I have any beer in the joint!"	*joint, articulation*
	Examples:	arthral (arthr/al)—pertaining to a joint arthroplasty (arthr/o/plast/y)—plastic repair (surgery) of a joint arthrodesis (arthr/o/desis)—the surgical fixation of a joint	
-asthenia (as-the' ne-ah)	as the knee	It is a well known fact that disuse produces atrophy, and, in the leg, it can be seen as the knee that is the smallest is the one with the weakness, the one shrunk from disuse.	*weakness*

ELEMENT	MNEMONIC DEVICE	ASSOCIATION-IMAGE	MEANING
	Note:	This suffix combination is formed from three useful elements, the prefix a- meaning "not" or "lacking"; plus the root sthen- meaning "strength" or "strong"; plus the word ending -ia meaning "morbid (diseased) condition." Literally, the word can be translated as "a condition of lacking strength" or "weakness."	
	Examples:	adenasthenia (aden/asthen/ia)—a weakness in glandular secretion; deficient glandular activity asthenia (asthen/ia)—lack or loss of strength, energy asthenopia (asthen/op/ia)—a condition of weakness in the eye	
astr- (as'tro)	astronomy	Astronomy is the study of the heavenly bodies, some of which are star shaped.	*star shaped*
	Examples:	astrocyte (astr/o/cyt/e)—a star shaped cell, esp. nervous astroid (astr/oid)—star shaped	
aur- (aw'ral)	aura	Jody said, "I can only see her bright blue aura around her left ear."	*ear*
	Examples:	auricle (aur/i/cle)—the projecting part of the ear auris (aur/is)—the ear	
auto- (aw-toh)	ought to	Gloria said, "He ought to take care of his self, 'cause no one else will."	*self,* *self-caused*
	Examples:	autogenic (auto/gen/ic)—self-producing autopathy (auto/pathy)—a disease without external cause autoplasty (auto/plasty)—grafting from patient's own body	
benign (be-nine)	be mine	Be mine, *mild* or hot, for only love, not love me not, can serve us both.	*mild, not* *cancerous*
	Note:	The principal use of the word is to designate the absence of cancerous tumors as in "a benign tumor" versus "a carcin/oma."	
bili- (bill-eh)	Billy	Billy had a plan most vile, without a smile, the gall of him!	*bile*

ELEMENT	MNEMONIC DEVICE	ASSOCIATION-IMAGE	MEANING
	Examples:	biliary (bili/ary)—pertaining to bile or collectively to the bile, bile ducts, and gallbladder biliuria (bili/uria)—bile in the urine	
blephar- (blef-ar)	bluffer	One can often tell a poker bluffer by the twitch in his eyelids.	*eyelids*
	Examples:	blepharospasm (blephar/o/spasm)—involuntary movements (contractions) of the eyelid blepharitis (blephar/itis)—inflammation of an eyelid	
brachy- (brack-ee)	break	The class took a short break before starting again.	*short*
	Examples:	brachy/meta—measurably short brachy/faci/al—low, broad face brachy/gnath/ia—abnormal shortness of the under jaw	
brady- (brad-ee)	Brady	Imagine watching one hour of the TV show The Brady Bunch in slow motion; almost hypnotic.	*slow*
	Examples:	bradycardia (brady/card/ia)—abnormal slowness of the heartbeat (usually < 60 beats per minute) bradyglossia (brady/glossia)—abnormal slowness of utterance bradylogia (brady/log/ia)—abnormal slowness of speech due to slowness of thinking, as in a mental disorder	
bucc(o)- (buk-ko)	buck	A burr under the saddle will very likely cause a horse to buck with nostrils flared and cheeks puffed as you fall on your nether cheeks; oh, the pain!	*cheek*
	Examples:	buccal (bucc/al)—pertaining to the cheek bucally (bucc/al/ly)—toward the cheek	

ELEMENT	MNEMONIC DEVICE	ASSOCIATION-IMAGE	MEANING
burso- (bur-so)	burro	Jacob put the pack sack on the burro with care, as Jenny the burro was skittish.	*sac (usually with a lubricating fluid)*
	Examples:	bursitis (burs/itis)—inflammation of a bursa bursopathy (burso/path/y)—any disease of the bursa	
calc- (cal-sik)	caulk	He filled the seam with caulk using the heel of his hand to press it firmly into the stone crevice.	*heel, stone*
	Examples:	calcemia (calc/emia)—excess of calcium in the blood calcic (cal/cic)—pertaining to calcium or lime	
cantho- (kan-tho)	can though	The angle at the end of my eyelid is not for me to see, but you can, though.	*angle at the end of the eyelid <o>*
	Examples:	canthal (canth/al)—pertaining to a corner of the eye canthus (canth/us)—name of the corner of the eye	

CHAPTER TWO

ELEMENT APPERCEPTION EXERCISE

Pronounce the word aloud, and then break down the word into its elements. Define the elements by stating the meaning of the last element first, then the others in order.

Example: Word = Auto/brady/asthen/ia = weakness, slow, self or a slow weakness of self. This word does not exist. Do you think that it could, or will in the future?

1.	abneural	20.	avulsion
2.	blepharalgia	21.	acoustics
3.	acroadenalgia	22.	aerasthenia[1]
4.	alveolalgia	23.	adenopathy
5.	adenosis	24.	adnexopexy
6.	algospasm	25.	algiomuscular
7.	alveolus	26.	ambisexual
8.	amebic	27.	amebiasis
9.	amphicrania	28.	amphodiplopia
10.	anesthesia	29.	bursoalgia (dynia)[2]
11.	angiomegaly	30.	antepartum
12.	anteroposterior	31.	abarthrosis[3]
13.	antigen	32.	antrodynia
14.	arthrodesis	33.	adenasthenia
15.	asthenopia	34.	antibrachium[4]
16.	autogenic	35.	biliuria
17.	brachygnathia	36.	bradylogia
18.	bursopathy	37.	calcemia
19.	canthal	38.	cantholysis[5]

---

[1]   Also Psychasthenia: Loss of self confidence and mental worry seen in pilots.

[2]   Dynia to be covered in later lesson. It also means pain.

[3]   Osis refers to "condition of", and is in Lesson Eight.

[4]   Brachium refers to the arm, esp. the upper arm.

[5]   Lysis—see page 64.

Meaning Point:

It must be understood that many medical words by direct definition do not carry a meaning identical with the roots or elements therein contained. When a word, such as psychasthenia does not seem to make sense, look it up.

CHAPTER THREE

MNEMONICS

ELEMENT	MNEMONIC DEVICE	ASSOCIATION-IMAGE	MEANING
capit-	capitol	The capitol of a state may also be the head of the state, some say the seat of the government; the latter may be significant today.	*head*
	Examples:	decapitate (de/capit/ate)—the act of beheading occipital (oc/cipit/al)—back of head biceps (bi/ceps)—two headed	
carcin-	car-sin	The preacher said, "Drunk driving is a car sin and a cancer on our society."	*cancer*
	Examples:	carcinogenic (carcino/genic) carcino-, a combining form meaning relationship to carcinoma; therefore, producing carcinoma carcinology (carcin/ology) oncology	
card- cardio- (kar-de-oh)	card	The card is the ace of hearts.	*heart*
	Examples:	cardiopathy (cardi/o/pathy)—any disorder or disease of the heart carditis (card/itis)—inflammation of the heart	
cata- (kat-ah)	catty	Catty remarks may be a form of condescension, a talking down to someone.	*down, under lower, complete*

ELEMENT	MNEMONIC DEVICE	ASSOCIATION-IMAGE	MEANING
	Examples:	catarrh (cata/rrh)—a flowing down; as in mucous catheter (cath/et/er)—"sending down" a tube into the body, such as a urinary catheter	
cau(s)- caut- (kawz)	cause	He said, "May the devil's fire cause you to burn eternally," but he was only reading a line from a play.	*burn, burning heat*
	Examples:	caustic (caust/ic)—burning or corrosive destruction to living tissue causalgia (caus/algia)—burning pain	
cauda- (kaw-dah)	caught a	He caught a fish with a very long tail; sounds like a fish tale to me.	*tail.tail part*
	Examples:	caudal (caud/al)—pertaining to the tail (the "rear end") caudate (caud/ate) having a tail	
cec- (seek)	seek	If a blind man seeks passage on a boat, does he seek a blind passage?	*blind passage*

The cecum (cec/um) is a large pouch at the beginning of the large intestine with only one opening. Additionally, the appendix hangs at the end of the cecum.

	Examples:	cecoptosis (cec/o/ptosis)—falling (downward displacement) cecitis (cec/itis)—inflammation cecal (cec/al)—pertaining to the cecum	
-cele (seel)	seal	Imagine looking at the ocean seeing one seal, then two more, then two more, riding on the ever-swelling waves.	*hernia, tumor or swelling*
	Examples:	myocele (my/o/cele)—a muscle hernia; protrusion cystocele (cyst/o/cele)—protrusion of the bladder through the vaginal wall	
celio- (see-leo)	see Leo	See Leo the lion, he's being taught to put one paw on his trainer's abdomen.	*abdomen*

ELEMENT	MNEMONIC DEVICE	ASSOCIATION-IMAGE	MEANING
	Examples:	celiac (celi/ac)—pertaining to the abdomen celitis (cel/itis)—any inflammation of the abdomen	
-centesis (sen-tee-sis)	sensitize	To immunize/sensitize it is often necessary to puncture the skin.	*puncture*
	Examples:	arthrocentesis (arthr/o/centesis)—into a joint cardiocentesis (cardi/o/centesis)—into the heart	
cephal- (sef-al)	self fell	For John, capital punishment was when his self fell hitting his own head.	*head*
	Examples:	cephalic (cephal/ic)—pertaining to the head cephalad (cephal/ad)—towards the head	
cerebr- (seh-ree-ber)	saber	The way he's spinning that saber one would think that he hasn't a brain in his head.	*brain*

cerebrum (seh-REE-brum)—the main portion of the brain occupying the upper part of the cranium, the 2 cerebral hemispheres, united by the corpus callosum, forming the largest part of the nervous system in man.

	Examples:	cerebritis (cerebr/itis) inflammation of the cerebrum cerebral (cerebr/al) pertaining to the cerebrum	
cervic- (ser-vik)	Sir Hic	Sir Hic, a knight in shining armor, often caught it in the neck while jousting; poor adjustment, I would say!	*neck or neck like structure*

This root is widely used in its form cervical and cervix:
cervix (cerv/ix)—used to name those parts of the large bones of the body where the bone becomes narrow behind the knob-like end (head). The narrow part of a tooth at the gum line is also called the cervix or "neck" of the tooth. The name is applied also to the narrow (constricted) parts of pear shaped organs such as the uterus and the gall and urinary bladder, cervical (cervic/al)—used to indicate a relationship to a cervix or to the neck as in the cervical vertebrae of the neck.

	Examples:	cervicofacial (cervic/o/fac/i/al)—pertaining to the neck and face cervicitis (cervic/itis)—inflammation of the neck of the uterus	

ELEMENT	MNEMONIC DEVICE	ASSOCIATION-IMAGE	MEANING
cheil- (kye-el)	Kyle	Kyle stood up when someone had said, "Shut up"; now he has a fat lip.	*lip*
	Examples:	cheilitis (cheil/itis)—inflammation of the lips cheilosis (cheil/osis)—condition esp. fissuring and dry scaling of the vermilion surface of the lips and the angles of the mouth	
cheir- chiro- (kye-row)	guy row	Joseph was watching a rowboat race on the lake and exclaimed excitedly, "Look at that guy row, his hands move so fast that you almost can't see them!"	*hand*
	Examples:	chiropractic (chir/o/pract/ic)—manipulation of the body, especially of the spine, with the use of the hands cheirarthritis (cheir/arthr/itis)—inflamation of the joints of the hands, including the joints of the fingers	
chole- (koh-lee)	cola	Richard's cola, after standing for an hour, became viscous and vile with a taste like bitter bile.	*bile*
	Examples:	cholecyst (chole/cyst)—the bile sac cholangitis (chol/ang/itis)—inflammation of bile duct	
chondr- chondro- (kon-drow)	condor	A condor must have great strength to maintain flight with powerful cartilage wing connections.	*cartilage*
	Examples:	chondral (chondr/al)—pertaining to cartilage chrondroma (chondr/oma)—a tumor composed of cartilage	
cilia (sil-ee-ah)	silly	John always raises his left eyelash when he makes a silly remark.	*eyelash*
	Examples:	ciliary (cili/ary)—pertaining to/resembling the eyelashes cilium (cili/um)—the eyelashes; also sometimes the eyelid, or the outer edge of the eyelid, or the edge from which the eyelashes extend	

ELEMENT	MNEMONIC DEVICE	ASSOCIATION-IMAGE	MEANING
cine- (sin-eh)	scene	It is the movement from one scene to another that creates a story during a movie; and your persistence of vision that creates image movement.	*move, movement*
	Examples:	cineradiography (cine/radi/o/graph/y)—motion pictures using X-rays cineangiography (cine/angi/o/graph/y)—using motion picture techniques to visualize blood vessels	
	Also:	kine- and kinet: kinesiology (ki/ne/se/o/logy) the science of the study of motion as it relates to human joint movement	
-clasis (klah-sis)	clashes	The two gangs chose to fight that day. It was the last of two clashes that would leave an aftermath of broken bones and destroyed property. A breakdown in communication was believed to be the cause.	*break, destroy*
	Examples:	osteoclasis (oste/o/cla/sis)—breaking a bone cardioclasis (cardi/o/cla/sis) literally a "broken heart"; actually, rupture of the heart	
colla (kol-ah)	cola	The cola being poured from the bottle pours slowly, like glue, frozen in the gelatin of time.	*glue, gelatin like*
	Examples:	collagenitis (colla/gen/itis)—inflammation of collagen fibers of connective tissue collagenosis (colla/gen/osis) collagen disease	
colpo- (kol-poh)	cold pew	Sitting on the cold pew I was at once aware of the hollow space beside me, where Virgina used to sit.	*hollow, vagina*
	Examples:	colpocele (colpo/cele)—hernia into the vagina colpocystitis (colpo/cyst/itis) inflammation of the vagina and the bladder	

ELEMENT	MNEMONIC DEVICE	ASSOCIATION-IMAGE	MEANING
contra- (kon-trah)	contradict	What Ed said was against and counter to the present system of belief, and a contradiction in terms as well.	*against, counter to*
	Examples:	contraction (contr/action)—acting against; a shortening, as in a muscle contraction contraindicate (contra/indicate)—indicate against	
cor (core)	core	He was rotten to the core, and that was the heart of the matter.	*heart*
	Examples:	cordate (cord/ate)—heart shaped cordial (cord/i/al)—simulating the heart The foregoing demonstrate another form, cord;—cardi- is most often used for conditions and therapeutic procedures; and coron-, meaning "crown", which is often used broadly to indicate the heart	
corn(e)- (kor-ne)	corny	The man with the horn is playing that old corny tune *Sweet Adeline*.	*horny, hornlike*
	Examples:	corn—build-up of thick horny tissue by friction or pressure corneal (corne/al)—pertaining to the cornea of the eye corneous (corne/ous)—hornylike or horny	
cost- (kost)	cost	The cost of the rib roast was too high, so I made time payments.	*rib*
	Examples:	costal (cost/al)—pertaining to, related to, or situated near chondrocostal (chondr/o/cost/al)—pertaining to rib and rib cartilage epicostal (epi/cost/al)—situated upon a rib	
crani- (kray-nee)	cranny	Once in the cave we began to look in every nook and cranny for the skull ☠ and crossbones, the mark of the treasure location.	*skull*

ELEMENT	MNEMONIC DEVICE	ASSOCIATION-IMAGE	MEANING
	Note:	crani- bony framework cephal- the head in its entirety cerebr- In the narrowest application, the cerebrum, the main part of the higher brain in which the higher mental processes take place; sometimes to denote entire brain and sometimes higher mental processes as in cerebration encephal- the entire brain psych- the mind, always the mental processes, never the anatomical parts	
	Question:	Where does the soul exist?	
-crine (krin)	crying	It isn't any secret, crying over spilled milk is a waste of time.	*to secrete*
	Examples:	crinogenic (crin/o/gen/ic)—stimulating secretion exocrine (ex/o/crine)—external secretion of a gland, as opposed to endocrine	
cryo- (kri-oh)	creole	The creole lady gave a piercing scream that shot a cold chill down my spine. It was time to run!	*cold*
	Examples:	cryotherapy (cry/o/therapy)—the use of cold hematocryal (hem/at/o/cry/al)—cold-blooded	
cut- (kyout)	cute	She is cute, but remember, beauty is only skin-deep.	*skin*
	Examples:	cutis (cut/is)—the skin cutaneous (cutan/eous)—pertaining to the skin	

CHAPTER THREE

ELEMENT APPERCEPTION EXERCISE

Pronounce the word aloud, and then break down the word into its elements. Define the elements by stating the meaning of the last element first, then the others in order.

Example: Word = Brady/cine/o/cilia = eyelash-movement-slow; or, a slow movement of the eyelash. This word does not exist, but it could!

1.	decapitate	18.	occipital
2.	carcinology	19.	cardiopathy
3.	catarrh	20.	catheter
4.	causalgia	21.	caudalward
5.	cecoptosis	22.	cystocele
6.	celiac	23.	arthrocentesis
7.	cephalad	24.	cerebration
8.	cerebrocephalocele	25.	cervicofacial
9.	cheilophagia[1]	26.	cheirarthritis
10.	cholangitis	27.	cholecystitis
11.	chondroma	28.	supercilium
12.	cineangiography	29.	osteoclasis
13.	collagenosis	30.	colpocystitis
14.	contraindicate	31.	cordial
15.	corneous	32.	chondrocostal
16.	craniad	33.	exocrine
17.	hematocryal	34.	subcutaneous

---

[1]   phagia see page 91

MEANING POINT:

The element cardia—also has the meaning of the cardiac end of the stomach. This will be important to remember for future lessons.

The prefixes: cor, cora; cord and core mean *heart; pertaining to the coracoid any long, rounded, flexible structure;* and *the central part of anything, such as the pupil of the eye.* When in doubt, ask, or go to the library and look it up!

NOTES:

NOTES:

CHAPTER FOUR

MNEMONICS

ELEMENT	MNEMONIC DEVICE	ASSOCIATION-IMAGE	MEANING
cyan- (si-an)	sayonara	Sayonara is such sweet sorrow; to bid farewell makes one blue.	*blue*
	Examples:	cyanosis (cyan/osis)—blueness condition, usually nail beds, lips, etcetera cyanuria (cyan/uria)—the passage of blue urine	
cyst- (sist)	cistern	A cistern is used to hold water. When small, it is sometimes made from an animal bladder.	*sac containing fluid, bladder*
	Example:	cystalgia (cyst/algia)—pain in the urinary bladder cholecystalgia (chole/cyst/algia)—pain in the gallbladder	
cyt- (site)	site	The felon's last living site was a prison cell.	*cell*
	Examples:	leukocyte (leuk/o/cyt/e)—white blood cell erythrocyte (erythr/o/cyte)—red blood cell	
dacry- (dack-ree)	daiquiri	Susan turned to face the now empty seat, tears burning her eyes, one even dropping into the daiquiri she held; but this too will pass, she thought, raising the daiquiri to two pouting lips.	*tear*

ELEMENT	MNEMONIC DEVICE	ASSOCIATION-IMAGE	MEANING
	Examples:	dacryoadenitis (dacry/o/aden/itis)—inflammation of a lacrimal gland (a tear gland) dacryocystectomy (dacry/o/cyst/ectomy)—excision of the wall of the lacrimal sac	
dactyl- (dak-til)	back' till'	It looked like he bent his fingers and toes back' till' they almost broke, but he was just showing off that he was double-jointed.	*finger, toe*
	Examples:	-dactylia (dactyl/ia)—a condition of dactyl/o/gram (dactyl/o/gram)—fingerprint	
dendr- dendro- (den-dro)	fender	He said that a tree jumped out and hit the car fender and it startled him; it was a shock to his nervous system.	*tree, branching (as in the nervous system)*
	Examples:	dendrite (dendr/ite)—name for the nerve fibers that extend from a nerve cell dendroid (dendr/oid)—branching like a tree or shrub	
dent- (dent)	dent	The dog's bite was definitely worse than his bark, as he left teeth marks indented in my arm.	*teeth*
	Examples:	dental (dent/al)—pertaining to the teeth dentiform (dent/i/form)—formed or shaped like a tooth	
dermat- (der-ma-to)	McDermat	McDermat pinched each coin to micro-thinness, why, even his skin was thin.	*skin*
	Examples:	dermatitis (dermat/itis)—inflammation of the skin dermatosis (dermat/osis)—any condition or disease	
-desis (dee-sis)	pieces	Visualize the pieces of a broken picture frame being fixed with glue and a binding with string.	*binding, fixation*

ELEMENT	MNEMONIC DEVICE	ASSOCIATION-IMAGE	MEANING
	Examples:	arthrodesis (arthr/o/desis)—surgical fusion of a joint pleurodesis (pleur/o/desis)—the production of adhesions between the parietal and the visceral pleura	
Homework Assignment:		Find at least three (3) more words ending with -desis.	
digit (dij-it)	dig it	There is something very soothing, I am told, about sand, especially when you dig it with your fingers and toes.	*fingers, toes*
	Example:	digital (digit/al)—pertaining to the digits (fingers or toes) as in a digital examination (done with the hands and fingers)	
dors- (doors)	doors	Eggbert was so angry, he left through the two back doors, slamming them behind him.	*back*
	Examples:	dorsal (dors/al)—pertaining to the back, or as reference to the "back side" from the front side by direction, et cetera dorsalgia (dors/algia)—back pain, pain in the back dorsolateral (dors/o/later/al)—pertaining to the back and side	
duct- (duck)	aqueduct	Jim created an aqueduct by using a long tube to bring the water from the ditch to the dry well; it was a long draw.	*tube, lead or draw*
	Examples:	abduct (ab/duct)—away from midline | → oviduct (ovi/duct)—a uterine tube	
dura (du-rah)	endure	Joe was aware of the hard times that he would have to endure.	*hard-dura mater*
	Note:	Used principally as a shortened form of dura mater, the outermost, toughest, and most fibrous of the three membranes (meninges) covering the brain and spinal cord.	
	Examples:	induration (in/dur/ation)—hardness, as in induration caused by the infiltration of an intravenous line epidural (ep/i/dur/al) located outside the dura mater	

ELEMENT	MNEMONIC DEVICE	ASSOCIATION-IMAGE	MEANING
-odyn (o-din)	dine	Allen took pepcid an hour before his meals so that he could dine without pain.	*pain*
	Note:	This word is really out of place here. Its actual form should be -Odynia.	
	Examples:	arthrodynia (arthr/odyn/ia)—pain in joint acrodynia (acr/odyn/ia)—pain in an extremity odynolysis (odyn/o/lysis)—loosening of pain, relief from pain	
dynam- (di-nam)	dynamic	He was a most dynamic speaker; his power to control an audience was something to see!	*power, force, strength*
	Examples:	adynamia (a/dynam/ia)—lack or loss of normal power; asthenia cardiodynamics (cardi/o/dynam/ics)—study of the heart's motions and forces involved in the heart's action	
dys- (dis)	disturb	Take notice of the sign on the bathroom door "do not disturb"; perhaps the room is out of order, and it's bad if you're in a hurry.	*bad, out of order*
	Examples:	dysacousia (dys/a/cous/ia)—hearing impairment where there is a distortion of frequency or intensity dysarthrosis (dys/arthr/osis)—also, dysarthria- deformity or malformation of joints—dysarthria: incorrectly applied to imperfect speech; stammering	
-ectasis (ek-tah-sis)	ecstasy	A feeling of ecstasy may cause one to inspire one's lungs to full expansion.	*expansion*
	Examples:	cardiectasis (cardi/ectasis)—dilatation of the heart angiectasis (angi/ectasis)—beyond normal stretching of a blood vessel pneumonectasis (pneu/mo/nectasis)—over-distention of lung tissue; emphysema of lung tissue	
-ectomy (ek-to-me)	act to me	He said, "The first act, to me, needs to be cut out, in part or all, if this play is to survive."	*surgical removal of all or part*

ELEMENT	MNEMONIC DEVICE	ASSOCIATION-IMAGE	MEANING
	Examples:	adenectomy (aden/ectomy)—surgical removal of a gland arthrectomy (arthr/ectomy)—surgical removal of a joint cardiectomy (cardi/ectomy)—excision of the cardiac end of the stomach	
-edema (eh-dee-mah)	demon- stration	The demonstration swelled hot with tempers on both sides, that only the fluid of time could quell.	*swelling by fluid*
	Examples:	pneumonedema (pneumon/edema)—abnormal amount of fluid in the lungs dactyledema (dactyl/edema)—abnormal swelling of fingers and toes	
	Question:	What does Oedipus mean?	
-emesis (em-eh-sis)	emcee is	Oh! My gosh, the emcee is vomiting all over the podium.	*vomiting*
	Examples:	emesis (eme/sis)—the act of vomiting emetic (eme/tic)—something that causes vomiting (drug) cholemesis (chol/eme/sis)—the vomiting of bile or gall	
en- (en)	pen	He has a pen stuck in his ear. Do you think that he's trying to scratch his brain?	*in, within, inside*
	Note:	Usually *em-* before b, m, or p	
	Examples:	empathy (em/path/y)—objective awareness of and insight into the feelings, emotions, and behavior of another person encephal (en/cephal-)—within the head, usually with reference to the brain	
encephal- (en-sef-al)	end self and all	If one puts a gun to his head, and therefore his brain, and pulls the trigger, one could end self and all.	*brain*

ELEMENT	MNEMONIC DEVICE	ASSOCIATION-IMAGE	MEANING
	Examples:	encephalic (en/cephal/ic)—pertaining to the brain; also, lying within the cranial vault encephalon (en/cephal/on)—name for the brain	
end- (end)	send	Please send them inside, they haven't the sense to get out of the rain.	*inside, within* *inner*
	Examples: Note:	endangium (end/angi/um)—inner lining of a blood vessel endocardium (end/o/cardi/um)—inner lining of the heart sometimes as ent—as in: entostosis (ent/ost/osis)—an abnormal growth within the medullary canal of bone	
enter- (en-ter)	entire	After gutting the pig, he had an entire wheelbarrow full of intestines.	*intestines;* *usually small*
	Examples:	enteric (enter/ic)—pertaining to intestines enteradenitis (enter/aden/itis)—inflammation of the glands of the intestines	
ependym- (ee-pen-dim)	pendulum	If one is to put a clock pendulum into storage it must be wrapped or covered.	*wrapping,* *a covering*
	Note:	Specifically, the membrane lining the cavities of the brain and the spinal cord.	
	Examples:	ependymal (ependym/al)—pertaining to the ependyma ependymitis (ependym/itis)—inflammation of the ependyma	
epi- (ep-ih)	epic	A TV series bases one epic upon another, in addition to being continued *ad infinitum* (ahd ihn-fee-nee-tuum).	*upon, in* *addition to,* *on, over, outer*
	Examples:	epidermis (epi/derm/is)—outermost layer of skin epicyst (epi/cyst)—over the bladder	
erythro- (eh-rith-row)	a wreath row	Kathie looked out of her window, and to her astonishment there appeared a wreath row of red roses along the walk to her house. It was spring!	*red*

ELEMENT	MNEMONIC DEVICE	ASSOCIATION-IMAGE	MEANING
	Examples:	erythralgia (erythr/algia)—a condition marked by pain and redness of the skin erythrocyte (erythr/o/cyt)—red blood cell	
-esthesia (es-thee-zee-ah)	he has the	He has the audience in the palm of his hand, and it's a good feeling; he's a sensation!	*sensation, feeling*
	Examples:	-esthetic (-esthet/ic)—pertaining to feeling anesthesia (an/esthes/ia)—condition of lack of feeling; usually regarding the production of anesthesia for surgery	
eu- (you)	you	He said to his dog, "Hi there, you are a good dog."	*good, well, normal*
	Examples:	eucholia (eu/chol/ia)—normal bile eukinesia (eu/kines/ia)—normal movement eupnea (eu/pne/a)—normal respiration	
ex- (ex)	exit	In order to get out and away from the burning building he had to use the fire exit.	*out, away from outside of*
	Note:	The element ex- may appear in several forms: exo- meaning outside, outward or outer exogenic (exo/gen/ic)—produced outside exopathy (exo/path/y)—disease originating outside the body extra- meaning outside or beyond extracardial (extra/cardial)—outside the heart extrahepatic (extra/hepat/ic)—outside of the liver ecto- situated on the outside; outside ectosteal (ect/oste/al)—outside of bone ectocytic (ecto/cyt/ic)—outside the cell	

CHAPTER FOUR

ELEMENT APPERCEPTION EXERCISE

Pronounce the word aloud, and then break down the word into its elements. Define the elements by stating the meaning of the last element first, then the others in that order ←.

Example: Word = dys-dactyl-o-desis = binding or fixation, digit, bad or painful binding of the digits of hands or feet. One could be more specific and state: cheirodysdactylodesis (this word does not exist).

1.	cyanosis	22.	Cyanuria
2.	cystalgia	23.	erythrocyte
3.	dacryoadenitis	24.	dacryocystectomy
4.	dactylogram	25.	dendroid
5.	dentiform	26.	dermatosis
6.	arthrodesis	27.	pleurodesis
7.	digital	28.	dorsalgia
8.	dorsolateral	29.	oviduct
9.	abduct	30.	induration
10.	odynolysis	31.	acrodynia
11.	adynamia	32.	cardiodynamics
12.	dysacousia	33.	dysarthrosis
13.	angiectasis	34.	pneumonectasis
14.	cardiectomy	35.	dactyledema
15.	cholemesis	36.	encephal
16.	endangium	37.	enteradenitis
17.	ependymitis	38.	epicystitis
18.	erythralgia	39.	anesthesia
19.	eucholia	40.	eukinesia
20.	exogenic	41.	extrahepatic
21.	ectocytic	42.	ectosteal

MEANING POINT:

[1]When you see chole/cyst together it usually means gall bladder.

Funnygrams: *Errors in interpretation of (usually dictated) medical terms.* (e.g., tending sheep for *tendon sheath;* funnel headed for *frontal headache;* B-9 tumor for *benign tumor;* sin awhile for *synovial;* can sell us for *cancellous;* and idiosyncrazy for *idiosyncrasy)*—to name a few. Can you think of any?
Write them below.

PRACTICAL EXERCISE IN THE STORY TEST

This is an exercise that you can do to practice your skill at deciphering from a story the medical terms taken from the first three chapters. In this test, you will find a short story-vignette made up of the association/images found in the first three lessons. There are eight (8) word elements to be found (usually you will have 10). Not all paragraphs will contain an association/image that refers to a medical word element. At the end of the story, put down in the appropriate paragraph number the medical word element that you believe has been indicated. Remember, the words that you put down are medical word elements, not lay terms. There is no answer sheet in this book. Before you have your first 100-element test this exercise will be covered in class. Again, if you have any questions, please bring them up in class.

BEAUTY AND THE ACE

1. There is a story told of a young lady by the name of Geraldine who needed money to pay off her mortgage. Somehow, she had gotten herself into a poker game with four men. We pick up the story after several hands of straight 5-card draw poker. Nothing is wild, except, perhaps, the fire in Geraldine's red hair.

2. Geraldine looked across the table into McDermat's eyes. One can often tell a poker bluffer by the twitch in his eyelids.

3. McDermat and Geraldine were head-to-head with the highest pot of the evening. All others had folded. The game was five card no draw, no peek; all cards face down, one card up before each bet. Ordinarily, in the card game of poker you ante-up with your bet before the cards are dealt. Then you can raise according to subsequent deals. In no peek, you put out an "ante", plus betting after each card is turned face up.

4. It was McDermat's bet. He had three aces and one queen showing. Geraldine had four kings showing. McDermat was betting that he had an ace down. McDermat pinched each coin to micro-thinness, why, even his skin was thin. Then he threw the coin into the pot. It was a 100-dollar gold piece.

5. McDermat's raise was too high. It was an unfair raise; he wanted her to fold. He was rotten to the core, and that was the heart of the matter.

6. McDermat mumbled to hisself, looking at Geraldine across the table, "She is cute, but remember, beauty is only skin deep."

7. Geraldine wrote out an IOU, placed it in the pot and turned over her last card. She delightedly stated, "The card is the ace of hearts!"

8. McDermat pulled a derringer out of his sleeve. A chill shot through the smoke-filled air. Then, he pointed the derringer to his own head and said, "If one puts a gun to his head, and therefore his brain, and pulls the trigger, he could end self and all!" What a poor loser.

9. Someone standing close to McDermat grabbed the derringer away from him, stating, "It isn't any secret, crying over spilled milk is a waste of time."

10. Well, as the story goes, Geraldine paid off her mortgage and McDermat never played another card game again, but instead, became a model citizen. So all is well that ends with the ace of hearts.

It is time to try your skill at completing this exercise by putting down the medical word element indicated in the story for each paragraph below. There are only eight. Allow yourself about 15 minutes. Questions can be brought up in class.

Paragraph Number 1   _____

Paragraph Number 2   _____

Paragraph Number 3   _____

Paragraph Number 4   _____

Paragraph Number 5   _____

Paragraph Number 6   _____

Paragraph Number 7   _____

Paragraph Number 8   _____

Paragraph Number 9   _____

Paragraph Number 10   _____

NOTES:

In this section of the test, you will find a short story made up of the *association-images* found in your book. There are 10. Not all paragraphs will contain an *association-image* that refers to a medical word element. At the end of the story put down in the appropriate paragraph number the word(s) that you believe have been indicated. Remember, these words you write are medical word elements, not lay terms.

JOE'S ADVENTURE

1. I had just landed at the airport in Honolulu when I met Joe. We were both heading for the same destination—Southeast Asia—the next morning. I couldn't help but overhear part of Joe's conversation with his girlfriend. Violet cried, "Sayonara is such sweet sorrow, to bid farewell makes one blue."

2. Joe was aware of the hard times that he would have to endure But he bravely told her not to worry; he did not want her to know how he really felt about the trip.

3. Living conditions in the jungle were not going to be ideal, this he knew. Although an able combat veteran, Joe could not get far enough away from spiders, it was a real phobia.

4. After what seemed like an endless flight, we arrived in Saigon. I knew I was going to like Joe when he suggested we first visit the officer's club. We made our way to the bar for a drink. Watching us from a corner of the room was the most intriguing woman I had ever seen.

5. Joe commented to the bartender, "A cistern is used to hold water. When small, sometimes made of an animal bladder." The bartender was oblivious to the remark and passed us the cistern anyway.

6. The woman who had been watching us, came to our table. Joe was transfixed. Her name was Madelyn, she said, and she was Creole. She had come over a few months before to entertain the troops. However, she hadn't done any dancing lately because she was in such pain. Joe's ears perked up, he immediately knew his medical training would be put to good use.

7. Joe suggested, "I am sure I can help you. Just tell me where it hurts." Madelyn looked at us coyly and replied, "Said the spider to the fly, 'Enter my chamber and we shall see what cavity have thee!'" She led us to a back room and Joe went to work. He massaged her body with care; his hands seemed to know where each pain resided.

8. Music started drifting through the thin walls. I asked Madelyn who it was that played so well. She replied, "The man with the horn is playing that old corny tune Sweet Adeline."

9. Shortly thereafter we returned to the bar. An officer was standing on the bar spinning his saber, and he appeared to be quite intoxicated. I thought to myself, the way he is spinning that saber one would think that he has not a brain in his head; maybe no head at all if he was careless.

10. When she saw him, the Creole woman gave a piercing scream that shot a cold chill down my spine, it was time to run. I started for the door hoping that Joe would follow; Madelyn was already gone.

11. But it was not to be. The military training in Joe took over. He stood on the bar and soon had everyone's attention. He was a most dynamic speaker, his power to control an audience was something to see! I soon noticed that many people were laughing, even the officer with the saber. I thought to myself, he has the audience in the palm of his hand (for him it must be) a good feeling, he's a sensation!

12. Eventually things quieted down. It was early morning when we finally made our way to our quarters. I was exhausted. But even in my tired mind I knew that this was going to be an interesting tour of duty.

ANSWERS

1. _____
2. _____
3. _____
4. _____
5. _____
6. _____
7. _____
8. _____
9. _____
10. _____
11. _____
12. _____

In this section of the test you will find a short story made up of the *association-images* found in your book. There are 10. All paragraphs will contain an *association-image* that refers to a medical word element. Some paragraphs will have more than one. Minor changes in grammatical syntax have been made to the *association-images* to tell the story. At the end of the story put down in the appropriate paragraph number the word(s) that you believe have been indicated. Remember, these words you write are medical word elements, not lay terms.

THE PRINCESS IN THE TOWER

1. Being held captive in the castle tower by the wicked wizard Billy was the princess Ariana Billy had a plan most vile, without a smile, the gall of him. He wanted the princess for his bride, but she was in love with Sir Hic, and would not agree to marry Billy.

2. One morning Billy told princess Ariana that he had Sir Hic sealed up in a room in the dungeon. He told her that he filled the seams with caulk using the heel of his hand to press it firmly into the stone crevice, and that he would only set him free if the princess agreed to marry him. The princess was very upset and began to cry. Billy told her it isn't any secret, crying over spilled milk is a waste of time.

3. For two days and nights Sir Hic tried to escape his dungeon room, he felt like Bambi (the fawn) trapped, with a bamboo fence on both sides although Bambi was able to jump the smallest one to safety. His dilemma was different however. Sir Hic found a small crack in one wall and began to break away the wall. He thought, some say I am free because I can move around on both sides of my internal world of mind; left and right, as if in two ways of thinking. But, in order to escape, I must use my hands. I must escape and save the princess Ariana.

4. Three days had passed and the wicked wizard Billy went to Ariana; he again told her he would free Sir Hic if she would agree to marry him. Ariana would not agree. "Be mine, mild or hot, for only love, not love me not, can serve us both," said Billy. Ariana said, "You are nothing but a windbag, Sir, full of hot air." She knew in her heart Sir Hic would escape and save her.

5. Sir Hic, a knight in shining armor, often caught it in the neck while jousting; poor adjustment, I would say. Somewhat dingy, but he was in love with Ariana and vowed to save her from the wicked wizard. Slowly the wall was breaking away, all of a sudden with a very loud bang the wall gave way. Sir Hic found his way to the tower where Ariana and Billy were. The wicked wizard was no match for Sir Hic. Actually, it was Ariana who finished the fight when she crowned the wizard with a large metal goblet. Sir Hic had jousted poorly as usual. But love shall conquer the day—always.

6.   As Sir Hic and Ariana were leaving the castle she said, "You know, he was rotten to the core, and that was the heart of the matter." Once outside, and free once more, Sir Hic noticed his old dog waiting for him. He said to his dog, "Hi there, you are a good dog." Sir Hic, Ariana and the faithful old dog lived happily ever after.

ANSWERS

1.   _____

2.   _____

3.   _____

4.   _____

5.   _____

6.   _____

CHAPTER FIVE

MNEMONICS

ELEMENT	MNEMONIC DEVICE	ASSOCIATION-IMAGE	MEANING
fascia (fash-ee-ah)	facial	She's having a facial done with a sheet of special tissue, and its being held on her face by a band around her forehead.	*sheet, band, fibrous tissue*
	Examples:	fasciitis (fasci/itis)—inflammation of fascia fasciodesis (fasci/o/desis)—suturing a fascia to skeletal attachment	
fiss- (fis)	fistful	A roll of quarters makes a heavy fistful and will split your lip as knuckles cleave to your teeth with the crunch of traumatic mastication.	*to split, cleave*
fistula- (fis-tyou-lah)	fist	He threw his fist at my jaw. I ducked, escaping within a narrow margin the full force of the blow that may have given me an early passage to bedtime.	*pipe, a narrow passage*
	Examples:	fistulization (fistul/ization)—surgical creation of an opening into a hollow organ or between two structures that were not connected before fistuloenterostomy (fistul/o/enter/ostomy)—the operation of making biliary fistula empty permanently into the intestine	
furca- (fur-ka)	furry cat	Imagine a black, furry cat in an alley, eating with a knife and fork, he is fat and out of shape.	*fork shaped*

ELEMENT	MNEMONIC DEVICE	ASSOCIATION-IMAGE	MEANING
	Examples:	furcal (furc/al)—shaped like a fork, forked bifurcation (bi/furc/ation)—divided into two branches, a division, as in carotid bifurcation	
gangli- (gang-glee)	gangling	Not only was he a gangling boy at that awkward age, the poor boy also had knot-like swellings for elbows and knees.	*swelling, knot-like mass*
	Note:	General term for a group of nerve cell bodies located outside the central nervous system; also, ganglion of the dorsum of the wrist	
	Examples:	gangliocytoma (gangli/o/cyt/oma)—a tumor of ganglion cells ganglionectomy (gangli/on/ectomy)—excision of a ganglion	
Question:		How is a ganglion of the wrist removed/treated?	
gastr- (gas-ter) gastro- (gas-troh)	Casper	Imagine Casper the ghost with his sheet shaped like a stomach.	*stomach*
	Examples:	gastric (gastr/ic)—pertaining to the stomach gastradenitis (gastr/aden/itis)—inflammation of the glands of the stomach	
gemin- (jem-in)	gemini	Gemini was Allan's astrological sign, and he was an identical twin as well; coincidence or master plan?	*twin, double*
	Examples:	gemin- form denoting relationship to twins or pairs geminate (gemin/ate)—paired, occurring in pairs	
gen- (jem)	generous	A generous man might give away his original productions. Would you?	*original, production originate, produce*

ELEMENT	MNEMONIC DEVICE	ASSOCIATION-IMAGE	MEANING
	Note:	It is in the suffix form that -gen produces many medical terms; that which is produced.	
	Examples:	gene (gen/e)—the biologic unit of heredity genital (genit/al)—pertaining to the reproduction organs carcinogen (carcin/o/gen)—cancer producing osteogenic (oste/o/gen/ic)—producing bone	
geron- (jer-on)	groan	Jenny gave out with a groan as she looked into the mirror; there were many signs of old age creeping upon her. As one ages, gravity will have its way with you.	*old, as in old age*
	Examples:	acrogeria (acr/o/ger/ia)—old extremities, premature aging geriatrics (ger/iatr/ics)—that branch of medicine that treats all problems peculiar to old age	
gingiv- (jin-jiv)	Jim give	The teacher didn't see Jim give his gum to Joe, as he put it into his mouth before the teacher looked his way.	*gum tissue of the mouth*
	Examples:	gingivitis (gingiv/itis)—inflammation of the gums of the mouth gingivectomy (gingiv/ectomy)—excision of the gums of the mouth	
glom- (glom)	glum	A feeling of glum hung over them like black ball-shaped clouds.	*ball, rounded mass*
	Examples:	glomus (glom/us)—a small, round anatomical swelling made up of tiny blood vessels glomerulus (glomer/ul/us)—a tufted structure or cluster generally composed of blood vessels or nerve fibers; used principally to designate coils of blood vessels in the kidney	
glosso- (glos-oh)	glossy	Imagine a 3-D glossy photograph with a tongue sticking out at you.	*tongue*

ELEMENT	MNEMONIC DEVICE	ASSOCIATION-IMAGE	MEANING
	Examples:	glossal (gloss/al)—pertaining to the tongue glossodynia (glosso/dyn/ia)—pain in the tongue	
glyco- gluco- (gloo-ko)	glue KO'd	After that last punch, he was on the canvas, stuck to it, glue KO'd; sweet dreams, but not of sugarplums.	*sweet, sugar*
	Examples:	glycemia (glyc/em/ia)—sugar in the blood glycosuria (glyco/sur/ia)—abnormal amount of sugar in urine	
grad- (grad)	gradual	His life of fame was one grasped in gradual steps, taken ad lib without the passion of love, but with the cool calm of deliberation.	*walk, take* *steps by* *degrees*
	Examples:	-grade (-grade)—suffix indicating a series of steps graduated (grad/u/ate/d)—marked by a succession of lines, steps, or degrees retrograde (retr/o/grad/e)—going backward digitograde (digit/o/grad/e)—marked by walking on toes	
-gram (gram)	grand	Before him there was ten grand, an amount that he had to record in the books, and he would write it all by hand.	*write, record*
	Examples:	cardiogram (cardi/o/gram)—recording of heart action myogram (my/o/gram)—recording of muscle contraction/action	
gran- (gran)	Granny Goose	John put his Granny Goose potato chips on the bench next to him. Along came a fat person and sat on them. Now his chips are mere particles, almost a grain once again; poor John!	*grain, particle*
	Examples:	granul- (gran/ul-)—form denoting relationship to small particles granulation (gran/ul/ation)—as in granulation of tissue/wound	

ELEMENT	MNEMONIC DEVICE	ASSOCIATION-IMAGE	MEANING
gravid (grav-id)	gravity	The doctor said, "My dear, you don't know the true gravity of the situation; you're not just pregnant, but pregnant with triplets!" Now that's heavy with child times three.	*pregnant*
	Examples:	gravidity (gravid/ity)—being pregnant gravidocardiac (gravid/o/cardi/ac)—heart disease of pregnancy	
gyn- (jin) gynec- (guy-nek)	gym	Phillip was a little short in the mental department; he dressed like a woman so that he could go to the ladies gym and they would think he was just another female; maybe he's not so dumb!	*female, woman*
	Examples:	gynecoid (gynec/oid)—looking like a female gynecomastia (gynec/o/mast/ia)—excessive development of the male mammary glands	
hallux (hal-uks)	Hal of X	Justin Rousseau approached Hal of X, a very tall man, who was without shoes. Justin then noticed that he only had a big toe for a foot, and was without other toes. Could this be megapod?	*big toe*
	Note:	This is the medical name for the great toe. Also: hallucis, plural halluces, is a corruption of *hallus*, from the Greek, to leap. Another possibility is the corruption of the term *allex*, a term for thumb. Hallux Valgus: a term relating to displacement of the great toe as seen in a bunion.	
helio- (he-lee-oh)	helicopter	As the helicopter flew between me and the sun, it blocked the glare of light, allowing me to see his face clearly.	*sun, light, sunlight*
	Examples:	heliosis (helio/sis)—sunstroke heliotherapy (helio/therapy)—treatment of diseases by exposure to sunlight	

ELEMENT	MNEMONIC DEVICE	ASSOCIATION-IMAGE	MEANING
hem(at)- (hem-at)	him	The plastic surgeon had just cut into a bleeder and had blood all over him.	*blood*
	Note:	Examples of the element hem- which end with the letter "m" used in the form hemat:	
		hematology—the study of the blood hematoma—a swelling of blood	
	Note:	If a root begins with the letter "h," it will retain the "h" if it begins a word; however, if the root is preceeded by some other element, the "h" will usually be dropped.	
		Examples of the letter "h" being *retained* when the element hem- appears at the beginning of a medical term:	
		hemangioma—a tumor made up of blood vessels hematology—the study of blood	
		Examples of the letter "h" being *dropped* when the element hem- appears *within* the medical term:	
		cyanemia—a bluish condition of the blood hyperemia—an excess (more than normal) amount of blood	
hemi- (hem-ee)	Hemingway	I was about halfway through the book *The Old Man and the Sea* by Hemingway, when I noticed that someone had ripped out the last 10 or 12 pages—talk about being upset!	*half, half of*
	Examples:	hemialgia (hemi/algia)—pain on one side of the body hemihepatectomy (hemi/hepat/ectomy) removal by surgery of half of the liver	
hepat- (hep-ah)	heaped	As the butcher cut up the chicken, he heaped all the chicken liver into a separate pile.	*liver*

ELEMENT	MNEMONIC DEVICE	ASSOCIATION-IMAGE	MEANING
	Examples:	hepatic (hepat/tic)—pertaining to the liver hepatitis (hepat/itis)—inflammation of the liver (hep-ah-tye-tis)	
heter- (het-er)	Heather	Heather was her other name, quite different from the name Helga.	*other,* *different from*
	Also:	hetero- and -eter	
	Examples:	heteradenia (heter/aden/ia)—any abnormality of the gland tissue heterogenous (heter/o/gen/ous)—differing or opposite in structure myeleterosis (myel/eter/osis)—morbid alteration of the spinal cord	
histo- (his-toe)	history	She had a history of allergic coryza with much use of facial tissue to blow her nose.	*tissue*
	Examples:	histocyte (hist/o/cyt/e)—a tissue cell histoclastic (hist/o/clast/ic)—breaking down tissue	
hom- homo- -om- home/o/- (hoh-me-oh)	hominy	The professor turned and stated, "While each kernal of hominy may look the same, it is important to realize that no two things are exactly alike, and this is the basis for the semantic exercise today."	*same, equal,* *like* *resembling*
	Note:	The element homo- also refers to the biological class which includes man, as well as mammals such as apes and monkeys; within this class man is further classified as *homo sapiens*, "the wise one."	
	Examples:	homeostasis (home/o/stas/is)—kinetic equilibrium homohemotherapy (homo/hem/therapy)—treatment by the injection of blood from the same species	

ELEMENT	MNEMONIC DEVICE	ASSOCIATION-IMAGE	MEANING
hormone (hor-mon)	harmonize	It takes two, two at least, to harmonize, to excite and set in motion those rare sound waves that please the otonomic sensibility.	*to excite or to set into motion*
	Examples:	hormonic (hormon/ic)—pertaining to or acting as a hormone hormonotherapy (hormon/o/therap/y)—treatment with hormones	
hydro- (hi-drow)	hydrant	When that dog lifted his leg, I thought he was going to kick the water hydrant.	*water*
	Note:	*hydro-* may also appear as *hidro-* when referring to a sweat gland and as *hygro-* when referring to moisture	
	Examples:	hyperhidrosis (hyper/hidr/osis)—excessive sweating hygroma (hygr/oma)—a sac, cyst, or bursa distended with fluid	
hyper- (hi-purr)	high person	He certainly seems to be a high person, maybe aloof is a better description, a more-than-normal pain in the posterior.	*above, more than normal, excessive*
	Examples:	hyperalgia (hyper/algia)—excessive pain or sensitivity to pain hyperemia (hyper/em/ia)—excessive blood volume	
hypno- (hip-no)	hypnotist	The hypnotist gazed deeply into the mirror to practice his art, but alas, he put himself to sleep; was he boring or did he have good technique?	*sleep*
	Examples:	hypnotic (hypnot/ic)—inducing sleep, a drug anhypnia (an/hypn/ia)—insomnia, abnormal wakefulness	

CHAPTER FIVE

ELEMENT APPERCEPTION EXERCISE

Pronounce the word aloud, and then break down the word into its elements. Define the elements by stating the meaning of the last element first, then the others in order.

Example: Word = hydro/cyst/o/centesis = puncture, sac or bladder, water; or puncture of a sac or bladder full of water. This word does not exist. Could it describe a procedure?

1.	amphicarcinogenic	20.	brachycephalic
2.	acrogeria	21.	gastradenitis
3.	homeostasis	22.	gangliectomy
4.	glossodynia	23	fasciodesis
5.	fissurae Cerebelli	24.	fistulectomy
6.	gangliocytoma	25.	hyperhidrosis
7.	hemigastrectomy	26.	gingivitis
8.	geminate	27.	gynecomastia
9.	glomangioma	28.	glycohemia
10.	hemihepatectomy	29.	gravidocardiac
11.	hallux valgus	30.	heliosis
12.	hypnogenic	31.	hemialgia
13.	hypohemia	32.	hyperadenosis
14.	hypercholia	33.	hydrohepatosis
15.	hydrocystectasis	34.	hyperhidrosis
16.	histoclastic	35.	heliotherapy
17.	homohemotherapy	36.	bifurcation
18.	fistuloenterostomy	37.	gingivectomy
19.	hepatologist	38.	heteradenia

MEANING POINT:

-osis = condition or disease; most frequently used to indicate an abnormal or diseased condition; sometimes used in words not relating to disease such as in hypnosis.

If the word *glossodesis* existed, what would it mean?

CHAPTER SIX

MNEMONICS

ELEMENT	MNEMONIC DEVICE	ASSOCIATION-IMAGE	MEANING
hypo- (hi-poe)	typo	"A typo is beneath me; I'm not that deficient, you understand," she blurted, red in the face with anger.	*under, beneath, deficient, less than normal*
	Examples:	hypoadenia (hypo/aden/ia)—diminished glandular activity hypotension (hypo/tension)—lowered blood pressure	
hyster- (his-ter)	history	History has told us of great wombmates by one who utters to us hysterically; could this be true?	*womb, uterus*
	Examples:	hysteralgia (hyster/algia)—pain in the uterus (womb) hysterectomy (hyster/ectomy)—surgical removal of the uterus	
-iasis (i-ah-sis)	Isis	Isis is the goddess of the condition of fertility, which is the formation of and the presence of a fertilized ovum.	*condition, formation of, presence of*
	Examples:	cholelithiasis (chole/lith/iasis)—condition of bile stones amebiasis (ameb/iasis)—infestation with amebas, especially intestinal (amebic dysentery) bronchocandidiasis (bronch/o/candid/iasis) candidiasis of the respiratory tract	
infer- (in-fer)	infer	Joy did not wish to infer that the job of typing was below her, just that she did not make typos.	*below*

ELEMENT	MNEMONIC DEVICE	ASSOCIATION-IMAGE	MEANING
	Examples:	inferior (infer/ior)—situated below or located downward inferolateral (infer/o/later/al)—situated below and to one side	
infra- (in-frah)	infra dig	An infra dig is not beneath the ground, but beneath one's dignity.	*beneath*
	Examples:	infracostal (infra/cost/al)—beneath the rib(s) infrapsychic (infra/psych/ic)—below the psychic level, automatic	
inter- (in-ter)	interfere	If you interfere with an argument between two people, you may be among the injured.	*between*
	Examples:	intercilium (inter/cili/um)—space between the eyebrows interdigital (inter/digit/al)—space between fingers or toes	
intra- (in-trah)	introduced	Have you been introduced to the one within yourself? It could be scary!	*within*
	Examples:	intracardiac (intra/cardi/ac)—within the heart intracarpal (intra/carp/al)—within the wrist	
iris (i-ris)	arise	As I arise each morning, I often can see a rainbow of colors in the sky.	*rainbow (eye membrane)*
	Examples:	iridic (irid/ic)—pertaining to the iris iridectasis (irid/ectasis)—dilatation of the iris or the pupil of the eye	
iso- (i-so)	I saw	What I saw were two equal values in logic since they both agreed on at least one premise, and in a syllogistic way, this confirmed the outcome for me.	*equal, alike*
	Examples:	anisodont (an/iso/dont)—having teeth of unequal size or length isodactylism (iso/dactyl/ism)—condition in which the fingers are of relatively even length	

ELEMENT	MNEMONIC DEVICE	ASSOCIATION-IMAGE	MEANING

COMPARE WITH:

isometrics:	equality in measure or force	
isosceles:	equal sides, as in triangle with 2 equal sides	
isobar:	equal pressure lines on map	
isotope:	equal place	

-itis (i-tis)	it's	If it's a flaming pain, it's arthritis.	*inflammation*
	Examples:	gastritis (gastr/itis)—inflammation of the stomach carditis (card/itis)—inflammation of the heart cerebritis (cerebr/itis)—inflammation of the cerebrum angiitis (angi/itis)—inflammation of the vessels	
kerat- (ker-at)	carrot	imagine a carrot in the shape of a horn, a horny carrot.	*horny, horny tissue also: cornea of the eye*
	Examples:	keratoderma (kerat/o/derma)—horny skin covering hyperkeratosis (hyper/kerat/osis)—excessive growth of the horny layer of the skin	
labi- (lay-bee)	label	The perfume bottle label read "kiss me quick", and depicted large red lips pursed as if to entice one to kiss without restraint.	*lip, or liplike structure*
	Examples:	labium (labi/um)—a fleshy border labiology (labi/ology)—the study of lip movement in singing and speaking	
lacrim- (lack-rim)	lacking	He was found lacking when it came to crying; without a tear for his beer, and not of good cheer.	*tear, the tears*

ELEMENT	MNEMONIC DEVICE	ASSOCIATION-IMAGE	MEANING
	Examples:	lacrimal (lacrim/al)—pertaining to tears; sometimes lacrymal lacrimotomy (lacrim/otomy)—incision into a lacrimal duct	
lact- (lack)	galaxy	Our galaxy is also called the milky way.	*milk*
	Examples:	lacteal (lact/e/al)—pertaining to milk lactigenous (lact/i/gen/ous)—producing or secreting milk	
lal- (lal)	lull	His speech lulled his audience into what seemed a comatose stupor.	*speech, babbling*
	Examples:	echolalia (echo/lal/ia)—meaningless repitition of words bradylalia (brady/lal/ia)—abnormal slowness of speech that may be associated with a brain injury or disorder	
lapar- (lap-ar)	leper	A leper may have white bleached areas on his abdominal wall, as well as his arms and legs, during the first stages of the disease.	*abdominal wall*
	Note:	laparo- (lap-ah-ro)—a combining form denoting relationship to the loin or flank. Sometimes used loosely in reference to the abdomen.	
	Examples:	laparocele (lapar/o/cele)—ventral hernia (front) laparocholecystotomy (lapar/o/chole/cyst/otomy)—incision of the gallbladder through an abdominal section	
later- (lat-ter)	later	Set some time aside for smelling the the roses, it is later than you think.	*side, side of the body*
	Examples:	lateral (later/al)—towards the side; away from the midline lateralis (later/al/is)—denoting a structure away from the midline as in the Vastus lateralis (ref: the quadriceps extensor mechanism)	
leio- (lye-oh)	lie	Someone once told me that there were people who could lie in such a smooth way that you couldn't tell.	*smooth*

ELEMENT	MNEMONIC DEVICE	ASSOCIATION-IMAGE	MEANING
	Examples:	leiomyoma (leio/my/oma)—tumor composed of smooth muscle fibers, usually benign leioderma (leio/derm/ia)—abnormal glossiness or smoothness of the skin (smooth also refers to involuntary muscle)	
leuk- (luke)	Luke	Look, Luke is pallid, almost white.	*white-the color white*
	Examples:	leukocythemia (leuk/o/cyt/hem/ia)—leukemia leukoderma (leuk/o/derm/ia)—loss of melanin pigmemtation of the skin	
lien- (li-en) splen/o	lean	Seth became very lean after having his spleen removed, but he lived!	*spleen*
	Examples:	lienal (lien/al)—pertaining to the spleen lienitis (lien/itis)—splenitis	
lingua (ling-gwah) linguo- (ling-gwo)	lingo	Listen to the stranger's lingo; he speaks a foreign tongue.	*tongue* *(landmark)*
	Examples:	lingual (lingu/al)—pertaining to the tongue sublingual (sub/lingu/al)—under the tongue linguogingival (lingu/o/gingiv/al)—pertaining to the tongue and gums	
lip- (lip)	lip	John stood up when someone said, "shut up"; now he has a fat lip.	*fat, fatty tissue*
	Examples:	lipocardiac (lip/o/cardi/ac)—a fatty heart lipoarthritis (lip/o/arthr/itis)—inflammation of the fatty tissue of a joint	
lith- (lith)	lithium	Some say that lithium is a stone in the armamentarium of psychiatry; it sounds archaiac to me; perhaps they pushed the metaphor too far!	*stone, a calculus*

ELEMENT	MNEMONIC DEVICE	ASSOCIATION-IMAGE	MEANING
	Examples:	lithocystotomy (lith/o/cyst/otomy)—incision of the bladder for removal of stone(s) lithogenesis (lith/o/genesis)—formation of calculi	
lobo- (low-bow)	low blow	The reason that the fight was over was because one boxer gave a low blow to the other's mid-section.	*section*
	Examples:	lobectomy (lob/ectomy)—excision of a lobe, as of the lung, brain or liver lobar (lob/ar)—as in lobar pneumonia; pertaining to a lobe	
lumbo- (lum-bow)	Columbo	Is it true that Detective Columbo is now working on the *Case of the Sirloin Murder?*	*loins*
	Examples:	lumbocostal (lumb/o/cost/al)—pertaining to loin and ribs lumbodynia (lumb/o/dyn/ia)—lumbago	
-lysis (lye-sis)	lie,sis	He said, "There are ways to loosen your tongue, so don't lie,sis." Poor technique for a PI, don't you think?	*loosening, set free, destruction, release, decomposition*
	Examples:	hemolysis (he/mol/i/sis)—the breaking down of red blood cells litholysis (lith/ol/i/sis)—dissolution of calculi; stones in bladder	
macro- (mack-row)	make a row	The jolly green giant can make a row in your garden so large that you can drive your car in it, "Ho, Ho, Ho!"	*large, enlarged*
	Examples:	macrocephalia (macro/cephal/ia)—hypertrophy of the head macrodactylia (macro/dactyl/ia)—abnormal largeness of the fingers and toes	

ELEMENT	MNEMONIC DEVICE	ASSOCIATION-IMAGE	MEANING
macul- (mack-yule)	Mack	My friend Mack has a dog with many black spots; I think the dog is a Dalmatian.	*spot (or stain) specially of the skin*
	Examples:	macula (macul/a)—a spot or blotch maculation (macul/ation)—the condition of being spotted	
mal- (mal)	maul	I met a man on the road with a maul raised as if to strike, a bad sign, especially during the time when men wore, armor. But he was only waving hello, as those days are long ago.	*bad, abnormal*
	Examples:	mal/digestion (mal/digestion)—faulty or impaired digestion malformation (mal/formation)—abnormal formation, deformity	
-malacia (mah-la-she-ah)	malaysia	I had a friend once who thought people from Malaysia were soft and out of condition, until he met one.	*soft condition*
	Examples:	cardiomalacia (cardi/o/malacia)—softening of the heart angiomalacia (angi/o/malacia)—softening of the intima or walls of a vessel	

CHAPTER SIX

ELEMENT APPERCEPTION EXERCISE

Pronounce the word aloud, and then break down the word into its elements. Define the elements by stating the meaning of the last element first, then the others in order.

Example: Word = Angio/o/cerebr/o/malacia = softening, brain, vessel or possibly, softening of the vessels of the brain or both. Can you find this word?

1.	hypoadenia	23.	hypotension
2.	hysteralgia	24.	hysterectomy
3.	cholelithiasis	25.	bronchocandidiasis
4.	inferior	26.	inferolateral
5.	infracostal	27.	infrapsychic
6.	intercilium	28.	interdigital
7.	intracardiac	29.	intracarpal
8.	iridic	30.	iridectasis
9.	anisodont	31.	isodactylism
10.	cerebritis	32.	angiitis
11.	keratoderma	33.	hyperkeratosis
12.	labium	34.	labiology
13.	lacrimal	35.	lacrimotomy
14.	echolalia	36.	lateral
15.	laparocholecystotomy	37.	leiomyoma
16.	leukocythemia	38.	lienitis
17.	linguogingival	39.	lipoarthritis
18.	lithocystotomy	40.	lobectomy
19.	lumbodynia	41.	hemolysis
20.	macrocephalia	42.	macrodactylia
21.	macula	43.	maculation
22.	maldigestion	44.	angiomalacia

MEANING POINT:

Both—*algia* and—*dynia* elements mean pain; but it is often a matter of what sounds best when putting a word together. Obviously, *lumbodynia* sounds better than *lumboalgia* or *lumbalgia*.

Hypochondriac: The Latin term *hypochondrium* referred to the region below the cartilage of the ribs later designated as the abdominal areas below and behind the costal cartilages, on either side of the epigastrium. In these areas, various sensations of a distressing nature, were sometimes experienced without any organic disease being apparent. Considered to be due to a nervous complaint, such individuals have been called *hypochondriacs* due to the location of the disease; therefore, a morbid anxiety about one's health.

In this section of the test you will find a short story made up of the *association-images* found in your book. There are 10. Not all paragraphs will contain an *association-image* that refer to a medical word element. One paragraph will have more than one. To assist you on this test, you will find key words in bold relief. Minor changes in grammatical syntax have been made to the *association-images* to tell the story. At the end of the story put down in the appropriate paragraph number the word(s) that you believe have been indicated. Remember, the words you write are medical word elements, not lay terms.

A PUNCH IN TIME

1. John had always wanted to be a class fighter. He had started quite young. He also had a temper. After John burst into anger, it seemed that only ornery remarks came from his mouth. Once, John stood up when someone had said shut up, that got him a fat lip; and, was probably the reason he became a fighter in the first place.

2. John started his training at eighteen. His philosophy was: I always feel better when I am part of the labor force, for if I am not, I do not bring forth any bacon to the table.

3. After many preliminary bouts John was ready for the big fight. However, his first big fight ended quite unexpectedly. The reason that the fight was over was because one boxer gave a low blow to the other's mid-section.

4. After some time and a few more fights John got his big chance, a shot at the middleweight title. The fight started. After several rounds, he was not doing well and by the sixth round John was down for an eight count. He was the hometown hero and favorite, there was tension in the crowd, and a feeling of glum hung over them like black ball shaped clouds.

5. John was saved by the bell in the seventh round and while in his corner, he complained of right shoulder pain. His trainer said, "If it's a flaming pain, its arthritis." Some help he was!

6. Round eight found John quite tired. In the heat perspiration oozes from one who is in an overweight condition. Perhaps he had not lost enough weight or trained hard enough. It was a thought.

7. Round nine was John's downfall (literally). His opponent gave John a fierce blow to the apex of his jaw. After that last punch, he was on the canvas, stuck to it, glue KO'ed, sweet dreams, but not of sugarplums.

8. When John woke up, his trainer said, "Set some time aside for smelling the roses, it is later than you think."

9. Well not everything was bad, even though John had lost; there was a good purse to be had for the competition. Before John there was ten grand, an amount that he had to record in the books, and he would write it all by hand.

10. Our memory of John may have since faded, as do the memories of the many that challenge, but take no fame; but, within John's mind the memory of that fight will always be as fresh as yesterday. Sorry John, but fame is only for the very few.

ANSWERS

1. _____
2. _____
3. _____
4. _____
5. _____
6. _____
7. _____
8. _____
9. _____
10. _____

In this section of the test you will find a short story made up of the *association-images* found in your book. There are 10. All paragraphs will contain an *association-image* that refer to a medical word element. Some paragraphs will have more than one. Minor changes in grammatical syntax have been made to the *association-images* to tell the story. At the end of the story put down in the appropriate paragraph number the word(s) that you believe have been indicated. Remember, these words you write are medical word elements, not lay terms.

THE GREAT JOHN SULLIVAN

1. Drinking alcohol before any activity that requires critical thinking may be nulling to the mind, even harmful, producing bad outcomes in thinking. It only takes an evening at the local pub to show what I mean. Remember the night I told you about when we visited the pirate's cave? That ain't a patch on the night ol' John decided he wuz the great John Sullivan re-born!

2. John started tellin' us about it, but before ya kin shout "Gorgeous George," his speech lulled his audience into what seemed a comatose stupor. It wuz so bad Gina (Heather wuz her other name, quite different from the name of Helga) starts snorin'.

3. 'Bout that time John puts his Granny Goose potato chips on the bench next to him. Along comes a fat guy 'n' sits on them. Now his chips are mere particles, almost a grain again; poor John! His ego was of regal proportion, enlarged to the max, because he thought he wuz of royal descent as it were, bein' the great John Sullivan re-born. So he ups and calls the puir fat guy a blight and a bane and a blot on the name of all Irishmen.

4. In the thickest brogue ye've never heerd, the fat man sez, "Someone once told me there're people who could lie in such a smooth way, that you couldn't tell. I do believe he was a drunken Irishman as well." Ol' John comes back with, "He certainly seems to be a high person, maybe aloof is a better description, a more than normal pain in the posterior."

5. "'Tis enough ta bring a tear ta me eye, heerin' ya insult th' Irish that way," Sez John. We all knowed it wern't so, bein' as he wuz found lacking when it came to crying; without a tear for his beer, and not of good cheer, neither. "But the great Johnny Sullivan ne'er shed a tear in his beer, nor shall I," and up he jumps, swingin' and' a punchin'.

6. I starts up as well, thinkin' the puir fat man will need help, but then thinks ta myself, "Self, it you interferes with an argument between two people, you

may be among the injured; besides, ol' Johnny's so drunk, he's no real danger." Almost right, I wuz.

7.   Johnny had missed landin' any punch so far, but finally one connected. He starts up from the floor with a right, a real hay maker, and swings so hard he spins himself around, 'n' his jaw connects with his own fist, comin' round ta' other way! After that punch, he was on the canvas, stuck to it, glue KO'd, sweet dreams, but not of sugar plums, he be a' havin'.

8.   The fat man busts out laughin' 'n' falls off his stool, and the Crash! wakes up Heather (whose other name is Gina), who jumps up hollerin' and trips over th' puir fat man. "Well," sez Gina, lookin' nose to nose with puir ol' Johnny, out cold as a landlord's heart, "Maybe dreams DO come true!"

ANSWERS

1.   _____
2.   _____
3.   _____
4.   _____
5.   _____
6.   _____
7.   _____
8.   _____

CHAPTER SEVEN

MNEMONICS

ELEMENT	MNEMONIC DEVICE	ASSOCIATION-IMAGE	MEANING
malign- (muh-lin)	nulling	Drinking alcohol before any activity that requires critical thinking may be nulling to the mind, even harmful, producing bad outcomes in thinking.	*bad, harmful*
	Examples:	malignant (malign/ant)—progressing in virulence malignancy (malign/ancy)—tending to spread and become progressively worse; also metastasis	
mamm- (mam)	mammal	A whale is a mammal; therefore, the female must breast-feed her young.	*breast*
	Examples:	mammose (mamm/ose)—having large breasts mammalgia (mamm/algia)—pain in the mammary gland	
mani- (main-ee)	mania	My main mania is not a madness, only a preoccupation with poetry and fiction.	*madness, mental disturbance*
	Examples:	hypomania (hypo/mania)—madness of a moderate type megalomania (megal/o/mania)—mental state characterized by delusions of exaggerated personal importance	
mast- (mast)	master	"To master breast feeding, one must first learn to relax," Sharon said with a slight blush.	*breast front of chest, rare*

ELEMENT	MNEMONIC DEVICE	ASSOCIATION-IMAGE	MEANING
	Examples:	mastitis (mast/itis)—inflammation of the breast or milk secreting gland mastopathy (mas-top-ah-thee)—any disease of the mammary gland	
maxill- (mack-sil)	Maxwell	Mr. Maxwell has a prominent upper jawbone that sticks out as he talks; what an overbite!	*upper jawbone*
	Examples:	maxillary (mack-sih-ler-ee)—pertaining to the jawbone maxillolabial (mack-sil-oh-lay'-be-al)—pertaining to upper jawbone and the lip	
mechano- (me-kan-oh)	mechanical	"When it comes to a machine, I'm just not mechanical at all," George said.	*machine*
	Examples:	mechanotherapy (mek-ah-no-ther'-ah-pee)—use of mechanical devices in treatment of disease or its results mechanism (mek'-ah-nizm)—to disignate a system or a mental or physical process by which some result is produced	
megal- (meg-al)	regal	His ego was of regal proportion, enlarged to the max, because he thought he was of royal descent.	*enlarged* *(abnormal)*
	Examples:	acromegaly (ack-roh-meg-ah-lee)—enlarged extremities cardiomegaly (kar-dee-oh-meg-ah-lee)—enlarged heart	
melan- (mel-an)	Melanie	Imagine a girl named Melanie wearing black boots and saying, "These boots are made for walking . . . . "	*black*
	Examples:	melanocyte (mel-ah-no-sights)—the cell responsible for the production of black pigment melanosis (mel-ah-no-sis)—condition of unusual deposits of black pigment in different parts of the body	

ELEMENT	MNEMONIC DEVICE	ASSOCIATION-IMAGE	MEANING
mening- (me-ning)	meaning	The meaning of this element is membrane	*membrane, the membranes covering the brain and spinal cord (myel-)*
	Examples:	meningoencephalocele (me-ning-oh-en-sef'-ah-lo-seel) —hernial tissue through a defect in the cranium meningitis (me-nin-ji'-tis)—inflammation of the meninges with both mental and motor symptoms	
ment- (ment)	mint	His mind was in mint condition; but I am not so sure that is a positive statement these days.	*the mind*
	Examples:	mental (ment-al)—pertaining to the mind dementia (de-men'she-ah)—progressive mental deterioration due to organic disease of the brain	
	Note:	The preferred term use for mental processes is psycho- and psyche-	
metabol(e) (me-tab-ol)	met a fool	I met a fool along the path of life in my youth and that same fool along the path of old age; there was no change but time, I fear.	*change*
	Examples:	metabolism (me-tab'o-lizm)—the sum total of the physical and chemical processes by which an organism converts simpler compounds into living, organized substance. metabolite (me-tab'o-lite)—any compound produced during metabolism	
metr- (met'r)	matter	"The fact of the matter is that if you tear us apart, it will take more than love or money because we are wombmates and Siamese twins," they said simultaneously.	*uterus (womb)*

ELEMENT	MNEMONIC DEVICE	ASSOCIATION-IMAGE	MEANING
	Examples:	metrodynia (me-troh-din-ee-ah)—pain in the uterus endometrium (en-doe-metree-um)—the mucous coat (lining) of the uterus	
micr- (mike-r)	microbe	A microbe is a plant or animal so small that it can only be seen through a microscope	*small in size*
	Examples:	micrencephaly (mike-kren-sef'-ah-lee)—abnormal smallness and underdevelopment of the brain (micrencephalous) microadenopathy (mike-crow-aden-op-ah-thee)—disease of the small lymphatics	
my- (my)	my gosh	"My gosh," he said, "Did you see the size of *her* upper arm muscle?"	*muscle*
	Examples:	angiomyoma (an-jee-oh-my-oh-ma)—tumor consisting of blood and muscle elements myogenic (my-oh-jen-ik)—producing muscle fibers and muscles	
myco- (my-ko)	my comb	After a month in the jungle my comb had fungus all over it.	*fungus*
	Examples:	dermatomycosis (der-mat-toe-my-co-sis)—fungus infection of the skin acromycosis (ack-roe-my-co-sis)—fungus of the extremities	
myel- ((my-el)	mile	The doctor came at me with the spinal tap needle, and it looked a mile long. I said, "Could we do this to*marrow*!!"	*marrow* *(spinal cord)*
	Examples:	osteomyelitis (oss-tee-oh-my-eh-lye-tis)—inflammation of bone and bone marrow myelosis (my-eh-loh-sis)—means a tumor of the spinal cord and also an abnormal proliferation of bone marrow tissue	
myring- (my-ring)	my ring	My ring is an earring with a little drum hanging down.	*eardrum* *(tympanic membrane)*

ELEMENT	MNEMONIC DEVICE	ASSOCIATION-IMAGE	MEANING
	Examples:	myringitis (mir-in-jigh-tis)—inflammation of the eardrum myringotomy (mir-in-got-oh-me)—incision of eardrum to drain fluid	
neo- (nee-oh)	kneehole	George looked down at his jeans; working on his knees had created a new kneehole, it was time for patches.	*new, recent*
	Examples:	neo-arthrosis (nee-oh-ar-throh-sis)—false joint (nearthrosis) neogenesis (nee-oh-jen'-eh-sis)—tissue regeneration	
nephr- (nef-er)	never	"Have you never eaten kidney stew?" she said, stirring the pot.	*kidney*
	Examples:	nephritis (neh-fry-tis)—inflammation of the kidney nephrosis (neh-froh-sis)—any kidney disease, particularly marked by degenerative lesions of the renal tubules	
neuro- (nu-ro)	narrow	"Driving on a narrow road makes some people nervous; I think that I have more nerve than that," Sue said, holding the steering wheel tightly.	*nerve or nervous system*
	Examples:	neurosis (new-roh-sis)—mental disorder without any demonstrable organic basis neurocardiac (new-roh-kard-ee-ak)—pertaining to the nerves of the heart	
ocul- (ock-you'l)	oh cool	"Oh cool," he said, holding one eye closed as he looked through the telescope at the eye of the storm.	*eye*
	Note:	ocul- form denoting relationship to the eye ophthalm- form denoting relationship to the eye opt- form meaning visible or denoting relationship to vision or sight -opia—suffix element denoting a condition of vision or sight opt- and -opia related to function of the eye, that is, vision or seeing	

ELEMENT	MNEMONIC DEVICE	ASSOCIATION-IMAGE	MEANING
		ocul- and ophthalm- relate to eye as a physical or anatomical organ ocul- is generally used as a landmark ophthalm- is generally used to designate conditions of the eye and therapy applied to the eye	
	Examples:	oculonasal (ock-you-low-nay-zal)—pertaining to the eye and nose extraocular (ecks-trah-ock-you-lar)—on the outside of the eye	
odont- (oh-dawnt)	oh don't	She said, "Please Doctor, oh don't pull my tooth!!"	*tooth*
	Examples:	odontogenic (oh-don-to-jen-ik)—originating in the teeth odontectomy (oh-don-teck-toh-me)—extraction of a tooth endodontics (en-doe-don-ticks)—that branch of dentistry that deals with the inside of the tooth, principally the pulp within the root canal	
-oid (oid)	void	"Your mind is a great void, resembling the vastness of outer space," Jake said, looking Joe directly in the eyes, glaring. Joe replied, "And yours liken to a vacuum it would seem; what keeps your ears from collapsing upon themselves?"	*like,* *resembling*
	Examples:	lipoid (li-poid)—like or resembling fat myoid (my-oid)—like or resembling a muscle	
olfact- (ol-fack)	old fact	It is a known old fact that smell brings about the most primitive recall.	*smell, to smell*
	Examples:	olfactory (ol-fack-toh-ree)—pertaining to the sense of smell olfactophobia (ol-fack-toe-foh-bee-ah)—morbid aversion to odors	
-ologist (ol-oh-jist)	hallow guest	Evidently the preacher was our hallow guest because he was a specialist *in* the study of religion.	*a specialist in* *the study of*

ELEMENT	MNEMONIC DEVICE	ASSOCIATION-IMAGE	MEANING
	Examples:	neonatologist (nee-oh-nay-tol-oh-jist)—of the newborn psychologist (sigh-kol-oh-jist)—of the mind; emotional problems cardiologist (kar-dee-ol-oh-jist)—of the heart dermatologist (der-mah-tol-oh-jist)—of the skin; integument nephrologist (neh-frol-oh-jist)—of the kidney neurologist (new-rol-oh-jist)—of the nervous system	
-ology (ol-oh-jee)	allergy	Dr. Snifton was an allergy specialist, one who is an expert in the study of allergens.	*study of, knowledge of*
	Examples:	pathology (pah-thol-oh-jee)—study of the nature of disease physiology (fiz-ee-ol-oh-jee)—the science dealing with the function of various parts and organs of living organisms	
-oma (oh-ma)	Omaha	Brad told them that he was from Omaha, Nebraska, and in two more days he would return.	*tumor, new growth*
	Examples:	angioma (an-jee-oh-ma)—tumor which tends to be made up of blood vessels blepharadenoma (blef-are-add-en-oh-ma)—a tumor of the eyelid consisiting of gland-like structures, a glandular tumor of the eyelid	
oment- (oh-ment)	moment	We live only in the present moment of time, covering the events of now.	*covering (of internal abdominal organs)*
	Examples:	omentum (oh-men-tum)—name of the membrane omental (oh-ment-al)—pertaining to the omentum omentectomy (oh-men-teck-toh-me)—removal of the omentum	
onco- (ong-koh)	encore	The stage performer had 2 encores, then two more and two more, as the crowd formed a mass around him, cheering.	*mass, tumor, swelling*

ELEMENT	MNEMONIC DEVICE	ASSOCIATION-IMAGE	MEANING
	Examples:	oncology (ong-kol-oh-jee)—the study of tumors arthroncus (ar-throng-kus)—swelling of a joint	
onych- (oh-nick)	eunuch (you-nuk)	The veterinarian was a eunuch; it had something to do with a lion's nails or claw. I dare not ask.	*nail, claw*
	Examples:	onychia (oh-nick-ee-ah) an inflammation of the nail bed, resulting in the loss of the nail onychomalacia (on-ih-ko-mah-lay-shee-ah)—abnormal softening of the nail onychomycosis (on-ih-koh-my-koh-sis)—fungus infection of the nail	

CHAPTER SEVEN

ELEMENT APPERCEPTION EXERCISE

Pronounce the word aloud, and then break down the word into its elements. Define the elements by stating the meaning of the last element first, then the other elements in the same order.

Example: Word = Micr/o/metabol/ology = The study of, change, small or it could mean: the study of small changes.

1. malignant
2. hypomania
3. mastopathy
4. mechanotherapy
5. cardiomegaly
6. meningoencephalocele
7. metabolism
8. endometrium
9. microadenopathy
10. myogenic
11. osteomyelitis
12. myringotomy
13. neogenesis
14. neurosis
15. oculonasal
16. odontectomy
17. olfactophobia
18. pathology
19. blepharadenoma
20. arthroncus
21. leukonychia
22. micronychia
23. metromelanosis

24. mammalgia
25. megalomania
26. maxillolabial
27. acromegaly
28. melanocyte
29. dementia
30. metrodynia
31. micrencephaly
32. angiomyoma
33. dermatomycosis
34. myelosis
35. neo-arthrosis
36. nephrosis
37. neurocardiac
38. extraocular
39. lipoid
40. neonatologist
41. angioma
42. omentectomy
43. onychomalacia
44. onychomycosis
45. hepatonephromegaly
46. meningocerebritis

MEANING POINT:

The root mamm—is mostly used to designate the breast as a structure or landmark. For example:

mammose—having large breasts

mammoplasty—plastic reconstruction of the breast

In this section of the test you will find a short story made up of the *association-images* found in your book. There are 10. Not all paragraphs will contain an *association-image* that refers to a medical word element. Some paragraphs will have more than one. At the end of the story put down in the appropriate paragraph number the word(s) that you believe have been indicated. Remember, the words you write are medical word elements, not lay terms.

HAL OF X

1. Once upon a galaxy, a long, long time ago—before the FAX machine—a space ship entered the milky way. Shrouded by a sunspot's electrical activity, it made its way to our planet undetected. This is a story about how misunderstanding saved the day.

2. Justin Rousseau, an anthropologist, was working in a dig in a desolate part of Egypt. With him, there was an assistant named Helga and a Dr. Sominia, an etymologist and physician. Their primary purpose was to study old writings, fossils and the such. They had been hard at work and had not noticed a tall figure observing them. With a start, Justin looked up—a shadow had given away the tall one's presence. The intruder spoke, "Ketum em Hal ahf ex, Ko etum ve isis?" Dr. Sominia looked up, "Justin, I think he's called Hal of X; seems friendly, go talk to him." Justin Rousseau approached Hal of X; a very tall man, who was without shoes. Justin then noticed that he only had a big toe for a foot; was without other toes. Could this be megapod—he thought?

3. Helga turned to Dr. Sominia, "Listen to the stranger's lingo, he speaks a foreign tongue." Dr. Sominia said sarcastically, "I know that, I am an etymologist, you know!" Helga thought to her self—boy, his ego was of regal proportion, enlarged to the max, because he thought he was of royal descent. And he certainly seems to be a high person, maybe aloof is a better description, a more than normal pain in the posterior.

4. Justin was standing looking up at Hal of X. Hal of X repeated, "Ko etum ve isis?" Justin mumbled to him self; Isis is the goddess of the condition of fertility which is the formation of and the presence of a fertilized ovum. By that time, Dr. Sominia was trying to get Hal of X's attention by stating, "Our galaxy is also called the milky way."

5. Helga came up alongside of Dr. Sominia, "Maybe he's from that small country, you know the one, where the people of the small country had a bone to pick with their emperor that led to an oust. Maybe this is him?"

6. Dr. Sominia turned, "Shut up Heather!" Heather was her other name, quite different from the name Helga.

7. Justin turned to both of them and started to say something, but remained silent; if you interfere with an argument between two people, you may be among the injured.

8. Dr. Sominia listened to Hal of X, who by now seemed a little frantic, repeat his primary statement, "Ko etum ve isis?!!" Dr. Sominia scratched his head, "Are you from earth?" By this time Hal of X almost yelled, "Ko etum ve isis!!!" turned and ran off into the distance. Then, in the distance, a flash was seen. An object left earth in rapid time. Dr. Sominia turned to the others, "Someone once told me that there were people who could lie in such a smooth way, that you couldn't tell; I think this was the exception.

9. Well, thats how the day was saved. Many years later someone deciphered what "Ko etum ve isis" meant, which was, "Where is your bathroom?" Well, you guessed it, they, in their bumbling way, saved this planet from becoming an outhouse along the way to other stars and planets. Some say we are becoming one anyway.

ANSWERS

1. _____
2. _____
3. _____
4. _____
5. _____
6. _____
7. _____
8. _____
9. _____

In this section of the test you will find a short story made up of the *association-images* found in your book. There are 12. Not all paragraphs will contain an *association-image* that refer to a medical word element. One paragraph will have more than one. Minor changes in grammatical syntax have been made to the *association-images* to tell the story. At the end of the story put down in the appropriate paragraph number the word(s) that you believe have been indicated. Remember, these words you write are medical word elements, not lay terms.

All's Well With Maxwell's End

1. A generous man might give away his original productions, would you? This is a story of one who did.

2. He was a very gifted person, but not a handsome man. Mr. Maxwell had a prominent upper jawbone that stuck out when he talked; what an overbite.

3. He was a great composer and had many exciting performances. His life of fame was one grasped in gradual steps, taken ad lib without the passion of love, but with the cool calm of deliberation. He loved his music and loved creating a passionate response in his audiences.

4. Mr. Maxwell, through his experiences with his productions knew that it takes two. It takes two, two at least, to harmonize, to excite and set in motion those rare sound waves that please the otonomic sensibility. He only found true harmony twice in his life, once when he was young, when he thought he knew everything, and then again, when he was much older and much wiser. Unfortunately, it was true harmony between Luke and John. These two hated each other and constantly fought.

5. One time Luke told John to shut up. John stood up when Luke said shut up, and now he has a fat lip. But John got Luke back by punching him in the stomach. As Luke fell over, someone said, "Look, Luke is pallid, almost white!"

6. Mr. Maxwell sighed. A feeling of glum hung over him like black ball shaped clouds. He knew just how harmonious these two could be. So he sat down to talk. John said, "he threw his fist at my jaw, I ducked, escaping within a narrow margin the full force of the blow that may have given me an early passage to bedtime." Luke responded, "The reason that the fight was over was because he gave me a low blow to my midsection."

7. Being old and wise, Mr. Maxwell said to the two young men, "I met a fool along the path of my youth and that same fool along the path of old age; there was

no change but time I fear. I was that fool, and unfortunately, I did not learn. I have always regretted that. Luke and John . . . don't be fools. The two of you could have perfect harmony, don't give up the fame and fortune that I did just over some simple differences."

8. John and Luke decided that Mr. Maxwell was right and then and there made a truce.

9. Later that night the two of them with Mr. Maxwell leading gave the performance of their lives. The stage performers had 2 encores, and then 2 more and 2 more as the crowd formed a mass around them, cheering. Mr. Maxwell gave away an original production that night.

10. He remembered a time when he was young when he told another great composer, "If you interfere with an argument between two people, you may be among the injured." Unfortunately, he was not so wise then. But that is another story.

ANSWERS

1. _____
2. _____
3. _____
4. _____
5. _____
6. _____
7. _____
8. _____
9. _____
10. _____

CHAPTER EIGHT

MNEMONICS

ELEMENT	MNEMONIC DEVICE	ASSOCIATION-IMAGE	MEANING
oophor- (oh-of-or)	offer	Sam, the frying pan man, will offer you eggs overly done if you don't tell him how you want them.	*ovary*
	Examples:	oophoritis (oh-of-oh-rye-tis)—inflammation of an ovary oophorectomy (oh-of-oh-reck-toh-me)—surgical removal of an ovary	
ophthalm- (ahf-thalm) opt-	of film	He spied a film out of the corner of his eye, a roll of film not yet developed, unseen by any eyes, latent and waiting.	*eye or eyes*
	Examples:	ophthalmia (ahf-thal-me-ah) severe inflammation of the eye hemophthalmos (he-mahf-thal-mos)—extravasation of blood into the eye optic (op-tic)—pertaining to the eye optical (op-tic-al)—pertaining to sight	
or- (or)	ornery	After John burst into anger, it seemed that only ornery remarks came from his mouth.	*mouth*
	Examples:	orad (or-add)—toward the mouth orolingual (or-oh-lin-gwal)—pertaining to the mouth and tongue	
ortho- (or-thoh)	or throw	It wasn't normal for John to throw the ball straight, or throw it right to someone; no, he had to try throwing a fancy curve ball.	*straight, normal*

ELEMENT	MNEMONIC DEVICE	ASSOCIATION-IMAGE	MEANING
	Examples:	anorthopia (an-or-thop-ee-ah)—not straight vision, distorted vision orthopaedics (or-thoh-pee-diks)—branch of surgery dealing with diseases and injuries of bones, joints, muscles and tendons	
orchi- (or-kee)	orchestra	When I asked where the music students were, I was told that they were in the orchestra pit taking musical tests.	*testis*
	Examples:	orchiectomy (or-kee-eck-toh-me)—surgical removal orchitis (or-kye-tis)—inflammation of the testis	
-osis (oh-sis)	oozes	In the heat, perspiration oozes from one who is in an overweight condition.	*condition or disease*
	Examples:	gastrosis (gas-troh-sis)—a condition of the stomach dermatosis (derm-ah-toe-sis)—a condition of the skin	
osmo- (oz-mo)	osmosis	The rancid odor seeped through, as if by osmosis, the wet cloth he held to his nose; but he proceeded anyway.	*odor, smell*
	Examples:	anosmia (an-oz-mee-ah)—absence of the sense of smell osmics (oz-miks)—the study of odors	
ost- osteo- (oss-tee-oh)	oust	The people of the small country had a bone to pick with their emperor that led to an oust.	*bone, bone tissue*
	Examples:	ostealgia (oss-tee-al-jee-ah)—pain in bone tissue osteomalacia (oss-tee-oh-mah-lay-she-ah)—abnormal softening of bones due to disease osteonecrosis (oss-tee-oh-nee-kroh-sis)—death of bone caused by an insufficient blood supply, infection, malignancy or trauma through a nutrient vessel	

ELEMENT	MNEMONIC DEVICE	ASSOCIATION-IMAGE	MEANING
-ostomy (ahs-toh-me)	oust to me	The emperor escaped from his country by creating an opening secret wall. He stated, "I overheard a conversation and it sounded like an oust to me—I had to flee."	*to create an opening*
	Examples:	gastroenterostomy (gas-troh-enter-ahs-toh-me)—creating an artificial passage between the stomach and the intestines enthercholecystostomy (enter-koh-lee-sist-ahs-toh-me) —surgical creation of an artificial passage between the intestine and gallbladder	
oto- (oh-toh)	photo	Imagine a photograph; it's a picture of an ear.	*ear*
	Examples:	otalgia (oh-tal-gee-ah)—pain in the ear otomycosis (oh-toh-my-koh-sis)—fungus infection of the ear microtia (my-kroh-she-ah)—abnormally small ears	
-otomy (ot-toh-me)	autonomy	The surgeon had gone too far: he defined autonomy as one who could cut into himself; that is, make an incision into his very own leg, just for practice.	*cut into, surgical incision into*
	Examples:	arthrotomy (ar-throt-toh-me)—surgical incision of a joint craniotomy (kray-nee-ot-oh-me)—surgical incision into the skull	
ovar- (oh-var)	oval	As I sat there looking at the egg, I became aware that it was round rather than oval.	*egg (female reproductive gland)*
	Examples:	ovariogenic (oh-vah-ree-oh-gen-ik)—produced in or arising from within the ovary ovariocentesis (oh-vah-ree-cen-tee-sis)—surgical puncture of an ovary	
pachy- (pak-ee)	patchy	The patchy fog was so darned thick he couldn't spy the land.	*thick*

ELEMENT	MNEMONIC DEVICE	ASSOCIATION-IMAGE	MEANING
	Examples:	pachydermia (pak-ee-derm-ee-ah)—abnormal thickness of the skin acropachy (ack-roh-pak-ee)—clubbing of the fingers (thickening) pachyemia (pak-ee-ee-me-ah)—thickening of the blood	
palpebra- (pal-pee-brah)	pal Peter	As I remember my pal Peter, he was the one with the very large eyelids.	*eyelid*
	Examples:	palbebration (pal-pee-bray-shun)—abnormally frequent winking palpebritis (pal-pee-bright-tis)—blepharitis	
pan- (pan)	pan	What an idiot! He's passing around a frying pan for *all* to offer donations. I hope that the minister is not offended.	*all, completely*
	Examples:	panhysterectomy (pan-hiss-tch-reck-toh-me)—removal of the complete uterus by surgery panhypopituitarism (pan-high-poh-pih-too-ih-tar-ism)—generalized insufficiency of the pituitary hormones, resulting from damage to or deficiency of the gland	
para- (par-ah)	parrot	Imagine two parrots, one beside you and one beyond, in the distance, flying towards you, and landing by your side.	*beside, by the side, beyond, to one side*
	Note:	Also: *wrong, faulty, disordered*	
	Examples:	paracystitis (par-ah-sis-tye-tis)—inflammation of the tissues around the bladder paralysis (pah-ral-ih-sis)—"faulty loosening" = (Gr. lyein) and therefore the loss of a body part either in sensation or the ability to move (also: see meaning point at end of this lesson) parosteal (par-oss-tee-al)—pertaining to the bone covering also: periosteal	
pariet- (pah-rye-et)	pirate	He was an outstanding pirate; he could scale a ten-foot wall, with sword in mouth. in ten seconds; or in a conversation, put his foot in his mouth in five seconds.	*wall, of organ-cavity*

ELEMENT	MNEMONIC DEVICE	ASSOCIATION-IMAGE	MEANING
	Examples:	parietal (pah-rye-eh-tal)—pertaining to the walls of a cavity parietitis (par-rye-eh-tie-tis)—inflamation of the wall of an organ	
part- (part)	part	I always feel better when I am part of the labor force; for if I am not, I do not bring forth any bacon to the table.	*labor, bring forth giving birth*
	Examples:	parturition (par-tyou-rish-un)—giving birth postpartum (post-par-tum)—after child birth or delivery	
path- (path) -pathy	bath	The dermatologist said, "taking a bath too often may cause a skin disease; at very least a rash, especially if a perfumed soap is used."	*disease, suffering*
	Compare:	pathos (pah-thos)—a quality, especially in literature, that arouses feelings of pity	
	Examples:	pathosis (path-oh-sis)—a condition of disease arthropathy (ar-throp-ah-thee)—any disease of a joint chondropathy (kon-drop-ah-thee)—any disease of cartilage	
-penia (pee-nee-ah)	Penny	In the *Incredible Shrinking Woman* story, Penny grew smaller by a decrease in size daily.	*decrease, deficiency*
	Examples:	cytopenia (site-oh-pee-nee-ah)—deficiency of the cellular elements of the body hydropenia (hi-dro-pee-nee-ah)—deficiency of water in the body	
peps-,pept- (peps) -pepsia	peptobismol	If you attempt to digest too much too fast, you may need Peptobismol.	*digest, digestion*
	Examples:	dyspepsia (dis-pep-see-ah)—indigestion peptic (pep-tic)—pertaining to digestion	

ELEMENT	MNEMONIC DEVICE	ASSOCIATION-IMAGE	MEANING
peri- (per-ee)	Perry	Uncle Perry is quite large about his waist, it must be 60 inches around him at least; why, he is Mr. 5'x5'.	*about, around enclosing, covering*
	Examples:	pericardiocentesis (per-ih-kar-dee-oh-sen-tee-sis)—is drawing of fluid from the pericardial sac periodontitis (per-ee-oh-don-tye-tis)—inflammation of the gingiva and other tissues of the periodontium	
-pexy (peck-see)	sexy	The sexy stripper took too much off and now the show is up for suspension and she's in a real fix with the law.	*suspension, fixation*
	Examples:	nephropexy (nef-roh-peck-see)—is the surgical fixation of a floating kidney gastropexy (gas-troh-peck-see)—surgical fixation of the stomach	
phage (fage)	page	Pat was so hungry that he began to eat a page from the menu—boy, was the service slow.	*to eat, swallowing*
	Examples:	phagocytosis (fag-oh-sigh-toh-sis)—process of cells being engulfed by leukocytes (esp. diseased cells) odynophagia (oh-dine-oh-fay-gee-ah)—pain in swallowing	
phak- (fak)	fact	It is a fact that your eyes act as if they had lenses of glass, but they do not.	*lens of the eye*
	Examples:	phakitis (fah-kye-tis)—inflammation of the lens of the eyes phakoma (fah-ko-ma)—an occasional small, grayish white tumor seen microscopically in the retina in tuberous sclerosis	
pharmac- (far-mack)	pharmacy	A pharmacy is the new name for the old drug store of yesteryear.	*drug, medicine*

ELEMENT	MNEMONIC DEVICE	ASSOCIATION-IMAGE	MEANING
	Examples:	pharmacopsychosis (far-ma-ko-sye-ko-sis)—a term for any one of the group of mental diseases due to alcohol, drugs, or poison photopharmacology (foe-toe-far-ma-kol-oh-gee)—the study of the effects of light and other radiations on drugs and their pharmacological action	
phleb- (fleb)	fib	When John tells a fib, I can always tell because he has a large vein in his neck that stands out.	*vein*
	Examples:	phlebectasis (fleh-beck-tah-sis)—a varicosity, a dilatation of a vein phlebotomy (fleh-bot-oh-me)—venipuncture	
phob- phobia (foh-bee-ah)	foe	A foe may be one to fear.	*fear, abnormal fear*
	Examples:		

1.	gerontophobia	old age
2.	aerophobia	air or drafts
3.	monophobia	being alone
4.	zoophobia	animals
5.	apiphobia	bees
6.	hemaphobia	blood, sight of
7.	pedophobia	children
8.	noctiphobia	darkness or night
9.	iatrophobia	doctors
10.	kynophobia	dogs
11.	lipophobia	being fat
12.	theophobia	God, wrath of
13.	thermophobia	heat or tropics
14.	nosophobia	illness
15.	triskaidekaphobia	the number 13
16.	toxicophobia	poisons
17.	xenophobia	strangers

ELEMENT	MNEMONIC DEVICE	ASSOCIATION-IMAGE	MEANING
phon- (fon)	phone	If you listen, you can hear both voice and sound coming from my disconnected phone.	*voice, sound*
	Examples:	phonic (fon-ick)—pertaining to voice phonocardiography (foh-no-kar-dee-og-rah-fee)—a graphic representation of the heart sounds and murmurs (recorded)	
phot- photo- (foh-toe)	photo	The photographer said, "Stand here in the light so that I may take your photo."	*light*
	Examples:	photalgia (foh-tal-gee-ah)—pain, as in the eye, caused by light photoerythema (foe-toe-er-ih-thee-mah)—redness due to the exposure to light (could this be sun burn?)	

CHAPTER EIGHT

ELEMENT APPERCEPTION EXERCISE

Pronounce the word aloud, and then break down the word into its elements. Define the elements by stating the meaning of the last element first, then the other elements in the same order.

Example: Word = Gastrohydropenia = decrease, water and stomach; or, it could mean: the decreased production of water in the stomach.

1.	oophorohysterectomy	23.	oophoritis
2.	ophthalmia	24.	optical
3.	orolingual	25.	orchiectomy
4.	anorthopia	26.	dermatosis
5.	anosmia	27.	ostealgia
6.	osteonecrosis	28.	osteomalacia
7.	entercholecystostomy	29.	gastroenterostomy
8.	otomycosis	30.	microtia
9.	arthrotomy	31.	ovariocentesis
10.	acropachy	32.	pachyemia
11.	palpebration	33.	panhysterectomy
12.	panhypopituitarism	34.	paracystitis
13.	parosteal	35.	parietitis
14.	parturition	36.	postpartum
15.	chondropathy	37.	cytopenia
16.	dyspepsia	38.	pericardiocentesis
17.	periodontitis	39.	nephropexy
18.	odynophagia	40.	phakitis
19.	phakoma	41.	pharmacopsychosis
20.	phlebectasis	42.	phlebotomy
21.	triskaidekaphobia	43.	phonocardiography
22.	photoerythema	44.	photalgia

MEANING POINT:

para [L *parere*, to bring forth, to bear] a woman who has produced young regardless of whether the child was living at birth.

para [Gr. *para*, beyond] a prefix meaning beside, beyond, accessory to, apart from, against, etc. In chemistry, the prefix indicates the substitution in a derivative of the benzene ring of two atoms linked to opposite carbon atoms in the ring.

CHAPTER NINE

MNEMONICS

ELEMENT	MNEMONIC DEVICE	ASSOCIATION-IMAGE	MEANING
phragma- phrag- phrax- (frax) (frag-mah)	fragment	The fence was made from stone fragments piled as high as six feet in some places. It must have taken years to build.	*fence, wall off*
	Examples:	diaphragm (die-ah-fram)—a wall of muscle between the thoracic and abdominal cavities; used in respiration urethrophraxis (you-ree-throw-frack-sis)—blocking (obstruction) of the urethra	
phren- -phrenia (fren-ee-ah)	friend	He's a friend of mine.	*mind*
	Examples:	phrenic (fren-ick)—pertaining to the mind; pertaining to the diaphragm (also the phrenic nerve, a nerve with branches spreading mostly over the lower part of the diaphragm bradyphrenia (bray-dee-fren-ee-ah)—slowness of mental activity such as initiative, interest, or speech, frequently accompanying encephalitis	
physio- (fiz-ee-oh)	physical	He's a real physical specimen because he communicates intimately with nature; meaning his body, not his mind.	*nature, the body*
	Examples:	physiology (fiz-ee-ol-oh-jee)—the study of the function of the body and its parts physician (fi-zish-un)—an authorized practitioner of medicine	

ELEMENT	MNEMONIC DEVICE	ASSOCIATION-IMAGE	MEANING
pilo- (pye-loh)	Philo	Philo was an ancient philosopher with long white hair.	*hair*
	Examples:	pilus (pye-lus)—a hair depilation (dee-pye-lay-shun)—the process of removing hair	
plak- (plack)	flak	He said, "Don't give me any flak, now," and she threw a plate at him.	*a plate, also* *plaque*
	Examples:	leukoplakia (loo-koh-play-kee-ah)—is a disease marked by the development of white, thickened patches on the mucous membrane tissue of the tongue or cheek dental plaque (den-tal plack)—a deposit of material on the surface of a tooth—precursor to calculus	
-plasia (play-zee-ah)	plaza	When a new plaza is built, it's a new development and indicates growth for the community, and more taxes too!	*development* *or growth*
	Examples:	hyperplasia (high-per-play-zee-ah)—abnormal growth, usually abnormal increase in the number of normal cells in the normal arrangement in a tissue dysplasia (dis-play-zee-ah)—means abnormal development or growth, especially of cells.	
plast- -plasty (plas-tee)	plastic	If one puts a hole in a plastic ball, one must then do some plastic repair.	*plastic repair,* *renewal of* *destroyed,* *injured or* *deformed* *tissue*
	Examples:	arthroplasty (ar-throw-plas-tee)—surgical repair or replacement of a damaged joint blepharoplasty (blef-ah-roh-plas-tee)—surgical repair (or reduction) of the eyelids	
platy- (plat-ee)	Patty	It was said that Patty had a flat affect; I thought "concave" to be more descriptive.	*broad, flat*

ELEMENT	MNEMONIC DEVICE	ASSOCIATION-IMAGE	MEANING

Compare With: plak-, plax-, plat——flat or broad like a plate, a patch or eruption

Examples: platypodia (plat-ee-poe-dee-ah)——flatfoot
platyonychia (plat-ee-oh-nick-ee-ah)——abnormal flatness and broadness of the nails

-plegia (plee-jee-ah)	plagued	He was plagued by stage fright to the point of utter voice paralysis.	*paralysis, a stroke a loss of power*

Examples: cardioplegia (kar-dee-oh-plee-jee-ah)——paralysis of the muscles of the heart
paraplegia (par-ah-plee-jee-ah)——the paralysis of both legs and the lower part of the body

pleura (ploor-ah)	plural	The plural of membrane is membranes; aside from the fact that it covers the *chest cavity* as a serous membrane.	*membrane that covers the chest cavity, side*

Examples: pleurisy (ploor-ih-see)——an inflammation of the visceral and parietal pleura in the thoracic cavity
pleurectomy (ploor-eck-toh-me)——the surgical removal of part of the pleura

plexus (pleck-sus)	complexes	Rudy had several complexes with an interweaving network of anxieties that abraded his conscious reality to the point of madness.	*braid, an interweaving or network*

Examples: brachial plexus (bray-kee-al-pleck-sus)——network of lymphatic vessels, nerves, and blood vessels in the brachial region (arm)
plexal (pleck-ahl)——pertaining to a plexus

pneum- -pnea (noom)	noon	In the noonday desert air, his lungs became so parched that he could spit fire; well—would you believe dust?	*lung, air*

ELEMENT	MNEMONIC DEVICE	ASSOCIATION-IMAGE	MEANING
	Examples:	apnea (ap-nee-ah)—the absence of spontaneous respiration pneumothorax (new-moh-thor-racks)—an accumulation of air or gas in the pleural space, causing the lung to collapse	
pod- -podia (poh-dee-ah)	sod	The trapper looked down at the loose sod where a big foot print had been made; could this be the footprint from megapod?	*foot*
	Examples:	podiatrist (poh-dye-ah-trist)—foot doctor podedema (pod-eh-dee-mah)—swelling of the feet by fluid	
poly- (pol-ee)	Polly	My parrot Polly has many bright colors—she is too much!	*many or much*
	Examples:	polyacoustic (pol-ee-ah-koos-tic)—"much sound," increasing or intensifying sound polymyositis (pol-ee-my-oh-sigh-tis)—inflammation of several muscles at once	
post (pohst)	postman	The postman (or person) came late; he was behind in time, because it was after his usual time of arrival.	*after, behind in time or place*
	Examples:	postnatal (pohst-nay-tal)—means the time after birth posthepatic (pohst-he-pat-ik)—situated behind the liver	
poster- (pos-teer)	posture	His posture needed adjustment since his back part was protruding.	*back part, behind*
	Examples:	posterior (pos-teer-ee-or)—means situated in the back. It also means on the back part of an organ. The term is also used to refer to the dorsal surface of the body. posteroinferior (pos-teer-oh-in-fer-ee-or)—situated behind and below	
pre- (pree)	free	The clown was giving out free cotton candy in front of the circus tent before anyone had a chance to buy it inside.	*in front of, before prior to, earlier than*

ELEMENT	MNEMONIC DEVICE	ASSOCIATION-IMAGE	MEANING
	Note:	*preposterous*—pre- "before," and post- "after," which, as the Germans say, "Puts the horse behind the wagon." That is absurd—but of course, that is what preposterous means: *absurd.*	
	Examples:	prerenal (pree-ree-nal)—situated in front of the kidney preconscious (pree-kon-shus)—not present in consciousness, but readily recalled into it	
pro- (pro)	prologue	A prologue to my book is a poem in front of the book that you read before you actually read the book.	*in front of, before front part of, favoring*
	Examples:	proencephalon (pro-en-sef-ah-lon)—the front part of the brain proptosis (prop-toe-sis)—downward or foreward displacement of an organ or part	
proct- (prock)	protocol	They said that his diplomatic protocol was not fit for man or beast, calling him an *anus equines*, or worse!	*anus*
	Examples:	proctectomy (prock-teck-toh-me)—surgical removal of the rectum proctopexy (prock-toh-peck-see)—surgical fixation of the rectum to some adjacent tissue or organ	
proli- (pro-lee)	parolee	He was single in prison and if it is offspring he be wanting, it's a parolee he must be becoming.	*offspring, production*
	Example:	proliferate (pro-lif-er-ate)—Latin—*proles*, offspring, plus *fero*, I bear. Thus, increase by reproduction (cf. prolific). In pathology, the term is used for an abnormal growth of tissue, the multiplication of cells. The term came into use about 1850.	
pseud- (sued)	sued	He yelled out loud as they hauled him away, "I'm being sued under false pretenses, I tell you!!"	*false, imaginary*

ELEMENT	MNEMONIC DEVICE	ASSOCIATION-IMAGE	MEANING
	Examples:	pseudomelanosis (su-do-mel-ah-no-sis)—pigmentation of tissues postmortem from blood pseudoplegia (su-do-plee-jee-ah)—hysterical paralysis pseudomamma (so-do-mamm-ah)—a structure resembling a nipple, or even a complete breast, sometimes found on ovarian dermoids.	
psycho- (sigh-koh) psyche-	cycle	If one experiences an up and down cycle of mood swings, it may be that he has a bipolar mind, called manic depressive psychosis or illness.	*mind, mental processes the process of thought judgement and emotion*
	Examples:	psychosis (sigh-koh-sis)—any major mental disorder in which impairment of mental function has developed to a degree that seriously interferes with insight, the ability to meet the ordinary demands of life, or the ability to maintain adequate contact with reality psychodynamics (sigh-koh-dye-nam-icks)—the science of human behavior and motivation	
-ptosis (toh-sis)	toast is	It is said that Salvadore Dali painted a picture where toast is soggy, drooping and falling; sounds like my breakfast.	*falling, sagging, drooping a downward displacement*
	Examples:	blepharoptosis (blef-ah-roh-toh-sis)—drooping of the upper eyelid nephroptosis (nef-rop-toh-sis)—also known as a floating kidney, is a prolapse of the kidney (*prolapse* means the downward placement or drooping of a body organ)	
ptyal- (tie-al)	tylenol	After dental surgery John was given tylenol with an antihistamine to reduce pain and saliva production.	*saliva, spit*

ELEMENT	**MNEMONIC DEVICE**	**ASSOCIATION-IMAGE**	**MEANING**
	Examples:	ptyalectasis (tie-ah-leck-tah-sis)—dilatation of the salivary duct ptyalogenic (tie-ah-low-jen-ick)—formed from or by the action of saliva	
puer- (pyou-er)	pure	Her portrayal of pure innocence was childlike, but not necessarily vestal.	*child, children*
	Examples:	puerperium (pyou-er-pee-ree-um)—the period of three to six weeks after childbirth until the uterus returns to normal size puerilism (pyou-er-il-izm)—reversion of the mind to the state of childhood	
pulmon- (pull-mun)	Pullman	Imagine a Pullman car shaped like a large gray lung; it must be a smoker.	*lung*
	Examples:	pulmometry (pull-mom-eh-tree)—measurement of lung capacity pulmonology (pull-mow-noll-oh-gee)—science concerned with the anatomy, physiology, and pathology of the lungs	
pyle- pyloro- (pye-loh-roh)	pile	Imagine a pile of people behind a metal gate, all trying to get through at the same time,—what a mess!	*gate, an opening*
	Examples:	gastropylorectomy (gas-troh-pye-loh-reck-to-me)—excision of the pyloric portion of the stomach pyloroplasty (pye-loh-roh-plas-tee)—surgical repair of the pylorus	
rachi- -rachia (ray-kee-ah)	rake	Imagine a rake standing on its end. It has many round projections and looks like a wooden spinal column.	*spinal column*
	Examples:	rachiometer (ray-kee-omn-ih-ter)—apparatus for measuring spinal curvature rachiplegia (ray-kee-plee-gee-ah)—spinal paralysis	
radi- (ray-dee)	Ray	Ray was always late, but I spoke anyway, "Are you ready yet, Ray?"	*ray, beam, spoke*

ELEMENT	MNEMONIC DEVICE	ASSOCIATION-IMAGE	MEANING
	Examples:	radiopaque (ray-dee-oh-payk)—a substance that does not allow x-rays to pass through it cineradiography (sin-eh-ray-dee-og-rah-fee)—recording of images as they appear in motion on a flourescent screen	
radic- (rah-dick)	ridiculous	The inspector said, "This crime is quite ridiculous; we'll have to get to the root of it soon!"	*root, origin*
	Examples:	radiculitis (rah-dick-you-lye-tis)—inflammation of the root of a spinal nerve, especially that portion of the root that lies between the spinal cord and the intervertebral canal radiculoneuropathy (rah-dick-you-low-new-rop-ah-thee)—disease of the nerve roots and the nerve	

CHAPTER NINE

ELEMENT APPERCEPTION EXERCISE

Pronounce the word aloud, and then break down the word into its elements. Define the elements by stating the meaning of the last element first, then the other elements in the same order.

Example: Word = pseud/o/poly/plegia = paralysis, many and false; it could mean many false paralyses or possibly hysterical paralysis.

1.	diaphragm	26.	urethrophraxis
2.	phrenic	27.	bradyphrenia
3.	physiology	28.	depilation
4.	leukoplakia	29.	hyperplasia
5.	dysplasia	30.	arthroplasty
6.	blepharoplasty	31.	platypodia
7.	platyonychia	32.	cardioplegia
8.	paraplegia	33.	pleurisy
9.	pleurectomy	34.	brachial plexus
10.	apnea	35.	pneumothorax
11.	podedema	36.	polyacoustic
12.	polymyositis	37.	postnatal
13.	posthepatic	38.	posteroinferior
14.	prerenal	39.	preconscious
15.	proencephalon	40.	proptosis
16.	proctectomy	41.	proctopexy
17.	proliferate	42.	pseudomelanosis
18.	pseudoplegia	43.	psychosis
19.	psychodynamics	44.	blepharoptosis
20.	nephroptosis	45.	ptyalectasis
21.	ptyalogenic	46.	puerperium
22.	puerilism	47.	pulmometry
23.	gastropylorectomy	48.	pyloroplasty
24.	rachimeter	49.	rachiplegia
25.	cineradiography	50.	radiculoneuropathy

MEANING POINT:

PHRENIC (Greek—φρην, the diaphragm) . . . In Homer, the use of φρην, is for the parts about the heart, even the heart itself. Later it was restricted to the parts between the heart and the liver, thus the abdominal diaphragm. As this area was generally considered the seat of the emotions, and was also very properly considered to have some association with speaking, the term öñçí came to have the metaphorical significance of the soul or mind, a sort of affective centre. Thus the word *frenzy*, which is derived from öñçí, originally had significance of an emotional disturbance, but became identified more and more with mental disturbance.

CHAPTER TEN

MNEMONICS

ELEMENT	MNEMONIC DEVICE	ASSOCIATION-IMAGE	MEANING
ramus (rah-mus)	ram	Imagine a ram with branches growing out of his head instead of horns.	*branch, a branchlike projection*
	Examples:	ramitis (rah-mye-tis)—inflammation of a root ramose (rah-mose)—branching, having many branches	
ren- (ren)	wren	A wren had fallen, and kids on knees came to help this poor bird fallen from the sky.	*kidney*
	Examples:	renal (ree-nal)—pertaining to the kidney; usually as a landmark renal colic (ree-nal koll-ick)—an acute pain in the kidney area caused by blockage during the passage of a stone (*nephrolith*)	
retro- (ret-troh)	rhetoric	When unsure of his rhetoric, a teacher may take a step backwards while talking.	*backwards, back; situated behind*
	Examples:	retraction (ree-track-shun)—the act of drawing something back retroversion (reh-troh-ver-shun)—the tipping backward of an entire organ	
rhin- rhino- (rye-no)	ryenosesirus	"When one refers to my proboscis, I want you to know that I call my nose my ryenosesirus; a thing of splendor and royal size,"—so spoke Cyrano de Bergerac.	*the nose*

ELEMENT	MNEMONIC DEVICE	ASSOCIATION-IMAGE	MEAN
	Examples:	rhinesthesia (rye-nes-thee-zee-ah)—the sense of smell rhinoplasty (rye-no-plas-tee)—plastic surgery of the nose	
-rrhexis (reck-sis)	wrecks us	One balloon to another: "What really wrecks us is one tiny pin; it causes us to break or burst."	*a breaking, a bursting a rupture*
	Examples:	angiorrhexis (an-gee-oh-reck-sis)—rupture of a blood vessel cardiorrhexis (kar-dee-oh-reck-sis)—rupture of the heart	
-rrhaphy -orrhaphy (or-ah-fee)	raffish	Joe's raffish comment caused him pain and the need for eight sutures.	*suture, suturing*
	Examples:	myorrhaphy (my-or-ah-fee)—suture of a muscle nephrorrhaphy (nef-ror-ah-fee)—the suturing of a kidney	
rug/o- (roo-go)	rogue	Jeff was a rogue, a con man, a slime ball; he was taking a check to the bank, one he had pilfered, but the bank would not cash it because it was wrinkled, folded and creased. How sad!	*wrinkle, fold, crease*
	Examples:	rugae (roo-gay)—irregular ridges or folds in the mucous membrane. In the mouth, rugae cover the anterior portion of the hard palate rugosity (roo-gos-ih-tee)—the condition of being wrinkled; a fold, ridge or wrinkle	
salpingo- (sal-pin-go)	sell bingo	If you don't believe in gambling, I guess you can't sell bingo cards for the church; I guess you'll have to watch the boob tube.	*tube, especially the uterine tube*
	Examples:	salpingo-oophorectomy (sal-pin-go-oh-of-oh-reck-toh-me)—excision of the Fallopian tubes and the ovary salpingopexy (sal-pin-go-peck-see)—fixation of a uterine tube salpingostomy (sal-pin-gos-toh-me)—restoration of the patency of a uterine tube	

ELEMENT	MNEMONIC DEVICE	ASSOCIATION-IMAGE	MEANING
sarc- sarco- (sar-koh)	shark	A shark may eat the flesh of its own kind.	*flesh, fleshy material*
	Examples:	sarcolysis (sar-koh-lye-sis)—disintegration of the soft tissues; disintegration of flesh sarcoma (sar-koh-mah)—malignant neoplasm of the soft tissue arising from supportive and connective tissue such as bone, fat, muscle, bone marrow, and lymphatic tissue	
schiz/o- schis/o (skit-soh) (skiz-soh)	schism	A schism can be a division of a group into two discordant groups; a split, at times, into two separate factions.	*split*
	Examples:	schizophrenia (skit-soh-free-nee-ah)—psychosis in which there is loss of contact with reality, especially in regards to logical thought process; a distortion of reality that may include: dystonic voices, false beliefs, and paranoid ideation schizonychia (skiz-oh-nick-ee-ah)—splitting of the nails	
scirr(h)- (skir)	scurry	In his scurry, John tripped and fell hard on his posterior—oh the pain!	*hard, relating to a hard tumor*
	Examples:	dacryadenoscirrhus (dack-ree-ad-eh-no-skir-us)—a hard cancerous tumor of the lacrimal gland mastoscirrhus (mas-tow-skir-us)—a hard cancer of the breast	
scler(a)- (sklehr-ah)	scary	Joanne told Rudy that it was hard not to be afraid of the scary movie *Alien*.	*hard, white of the eye*
	Summary:	dura—short for dura mater, the hard covering the brain and spinal cord. An exception of use: induration, a process of hardness, as in induration of the skin scirrh—used most exclusively to refer to hard cancerous tumors scler(a)—can mean hardness or be a reference to the white of the eye kerat(o)—also means hard or horny, and is used in relation to the epidermis, hair, and nails	

ELEMENT	MNEMONIC DEVICE	ASSOCIATION-IMAGE	MEANING
	Examples:	scleraderma (sklehr-ah-derm-ah)—an insidious chronic disorder characterized by progressive collagenous fibrosis of many organs and systems, usually beginning with the skin sclerokeratoiritis (sklehr-oh-ker-ah-toh-ir-ih-dye-tis) —inflammation of sclera, cornea and iris	
-scop- -scopy (skoh-pee)	hope	The preacher said to his congregation, hope is look to the future, an observeation the self makes.	*look, observe, reveal*
	Examples:	bronchoscopy (bronk-os-koh-pee)—examination of the bronchus microscope (mike-row-skope)—an instrument for observing small things; the addition of the ending—*e* that carries a meaning of "instrument" forms this suffix stem meaning	
sedat- (se-dat)	Sadat	It was said of Anwar Sadat that he had a calming effect when he spoke; a way to quiet the masses; to avert war.	*quiet, calm*
	Examples:	sedation (se-day-shun)—the act or process of calming sedative (sed-ah-tive)—an agent, such as a drug, that calms; nerve sedative; hypnotic	
semen (see-men)	see men	If you look beyond, you can see men spreading seed in the fields; ones fertile with organic enriched soil.	*seed*
	Examples:	seminal (sem-ih-nal)—pertaining to semen semenuria (see-men-you-ree-ah)—semen in the urine	
semi- (sem-i)	semi	The semi was only half loaded.	*half, partially*
	Examples:	semilunar (sem-i-loon-ar)—resembling a crescent or half-moon seminormal (sem-i-norm-al)—one-half normal	

ELEMENT	MNEMONIC DEVICE	ASSOCIATION-IMAGE	MEANING
sept- (sept)	slept	Joe's back was stiff, as he had slept on the stonewall that was a fence, with alley cats all night; do not ask why!	*wall, fence, a division*
	Examples:	septotomy (sep-tot-oh-me)—incision of the nasal septum septum (sep-tum)—a general term in anatomy used to designate a dividing wall or partition; usually when *sept-* is used with no other qualification, the reference is to the nasal septum	
sinus (sign-us)	minus	A sinus cavity is a hollow space minus dense bone, that causes the head to weigh less; better for your neck, right?	*hollow space, cavity recess*
	Examples:	sinusotomy (sigh-nuh-sot-oh-me)—surgical incision of a sinus pilonidal sinus (pye-loh-nigh-dal sigh-nus)—a suppurating sinus containing hair, occurring chiefly in the coccygeal region	
somato- (so-mah-toe)	tomato	Eating a tomato every day is good for your body.	*body, the body*
	Examples:	soma (so-mah)—denoting the body, as distinguished from the mind somatopsychic (so-mah-toe-sye-kick)—pertaining to both body and mind somasthenia (so-mas-thee-nee-ah)—bodily weakness with poor appetite and poor sleep	
somni- (som-nee)	some knee	After the operation on his knee, John said, "Boy, that is some knee; now it's asleep most of the time."	*sleep*
	Examples:	somniferous (som-nif-er-us)—producing sleep; -ferous is an ending meaning *bearing* or *producing* somnipathy (som-nip-ah-thee)—any disorder of sleep	

ELEMENT	MNEMONIC DEVICE	ASSOCIATION-IMAGE	MEANING
spas- (spaz) -spasia	space	Out in space there are black holes that pull and draw material toward and into them.	*pull, draw - contraction*
	Examples:	myospasia (my-oh-spay-zee-ah)—a spasmodic condition in which rigidity of the muscles is followed immediately by relaxation spasmophilia (spaz-mo-fil-ee-ah)—abnormal tendency to convulsions	
	Note:	Clonus: (Gr. turmoil)—alternate muscular contraction and relaxation in rapid succession.	
	Compare:	Tonus—look up the meaning.	
spasm (spazm)	space M	On the robot there was a button with the designation space-M; if you pressed it, the robot would imitate a seizure disorder with involuntary contractions. What a sight!	*involuntary contractions*
	Examples:	angiospasm (an-jee-oh-spazm)—spasmodic contraction of the blood vessels laryngospasm (lah-ring-goh-spazm)—sudden spasmodic closure of the larynx	
sphenic (sfee-nick)	Phoenix	I am told that the mythical bird Phoenix arose from a pile of wedge-shaped ashes.	*a wedge, wedge-shaped*
	Examples:	sphenoid (sfee-noid)—resembling a wedge sphenocephaly (sfee-no-sef-ah-lee)—a developmental abnormality characterized by a wedge-shaped appearance of the head	
spiro- (spy-roh)	spiral	When she reached the top of the spiral staircase she looked down at the coil of stairs below and became quite dizzy.	*coil, winding twisting*

ELEMENT	MNEMONIC DEVICE	ASSOCIATION-IMAGE	MEANING
	Examples:	spiroid (spy-roid)—resembling a spiral or coil spiro- should not be confused with spir-, appearing in words such as perspire, perspiration, aspiration, respiration. In these words, the element spir- means "breath" or "breathing"	
spondyl- (spon-dil)	spindle	Having stacked the thread spindles upon each other, Rudy noticed that they gave the appearance of a wooden spinal column, each vertebra stacked precariously upon the other, but without ligaments for attachment— precarious indeed!	*spinal column or vertebra*
	Examples:	spondylosis (spon-dih-loh-sis)—any degenerative condition of the spine spondylolisthesis (spon-dih-loh-lis-thee-sis)—the partial displacement of one vertebra over the one below it	
squam- (skwam)	spawn	Imagine many fish swimming up a river to spawn; they have many of their scales damaged from the long swim.	*scale, a platelike structure*
	Examples:	squamoparietal (skwa-mo-pah-rye-tal)—pertaining to the squamous portion of the temporal and parietal bone squamate (skwa-mate)—scaly, having or resembling scales	
steno- (steh-no)	steno-pool	I thought that I would take a dip into the steno-pool, but it was too narrow, and so cold that I probably would have contracted the flu or something!	*narrow, contracted constricted, close*
	Examples:	angiostenosis (an-jee-oh-steh-no-sis)—the narrowing of a blood vessel stenocoriasis (steh-no-koh-ree-ah-sis)—contraction of the pupil	
stoma- (stoh-ma) stomato-	stone Ma	Upon coming to the crest of the massive temple, the great stone Ma idol with its big red mouth looked down at Jake, as if to blow him away; but only dead silence pervaded the air.	*mouth or opening*

ELEMENT	MNEMONIC DEVICE	ASSOCIATION-IMAGE	MEANING
	Examples:	stomatology (stoh-ma-tol-oh-gee)—the branch of medicine, which treats diseases of the mouth stomatomycosis (stoh-ma-toh-my-koh-sis)—a fungus disease of the mouth	
strepto- (strep-to)	strep throat	Doctor Paul swabbed Jim's strep throat with a deft twist of the wrist.	*twist, twisted*
	Examples:	streptomicrodactyly (strep-to-my-kroh-dak-tih-lee)—camptodactyly (clawlike condition of hand or foot) in which the little fingers only are involved streptohemolysin (strep-to-he-moh-lye-sin)—the hemolysin of hemolytic streptococci	
strict- (strik)	strict	A person with a strict demeanor may have a narrow outlook on life, often seen in their facial expression with lips drawn tight together in a perpetual frown— a sour puss, one might say.	*to draw tight, narrowing*
	Examples:	stricture (strik-tur)—abnormal narrowing of a duct or passage stricturotomy (strik-tu-rot-oh-me)—incision of a stricture	

CHAPTER TEN

ELEMENT APPERCEPTION EXERCISE

Pronounce the word aloud, and then break down the word into its elements. Define the elements by stating the meaning of the last element first, then the other elements in the same order.

Example: Word = semi/pelv/ectomy = removal of, pelvis, and half or removal of half of the pelvis. (look up under hemipelvectomy)

1.	ramitis	26.	ramose
2.	renal	27.	renal colic
3.	retroversion	28.	retraction
4.	rhinesthesia	29.	rhinoplasty
5.	angiorrhexis	30.	cardiorrhexis
6.	myorrhaphy	31.	nephrorrhaphy
7.	rugosity	32.	salpingopexy
8.	salpingo-oophorectomy	33.	salpingostomy
9.	sarcolysis	34.	schizophrenia
10.	schizonychia	35.	mastoscirrhus
11.	dacryadenoscirrhus	36.	scleraderma
12.	sclerokeratoiritis	37.	bronchoscopy
13.	sedative	38.	semenuria
14.	semilunar	39.	seminormal
15.	septotomy	40.	pilonidal sinus
16.	somatopsychic	41.	somasthenia
17.	somniferous	42.	somnipathy
18.	myospasia	43.	spasmophilia
19.	laryngospasm	44.	sphenocephaly
20.	spiroid	45.	spondylosis
21.	spondylolisthesis	46.	squamoparietal
22.	angiostenosis	47.	stenocoriasis
23.	stomatology	48.	stomatomycosis
24.	streptomicrodactyly	49.	streptohemolysin
25.	stricturotomy	50.	septalsinusopathy

MEANING POINT:

Soma (Greek—σωμα, body) Homer used σωμα for a dead body, but later meant the body generally, either of humans or animals. *Somatic*—relating to the body.

Ren—is used principally as a landmark, i.e. a point of reference in locating other nearby structures, while the root nephr—is used principally to name conditions affecting the kidneys (diseases, symptoms, etc.) and other surgical procedures performed on the kidney.

CHAPTER ELEVEN

MNEMONICS

ELEMENT	MNEMONIC DEVICE	ASSOCIATION-IMAGE	MEANING
sub- (sub)	Subaru	The pileup on 101 involved a Subaru that had turned under a truck and was now beneath one wheel and under another.	*under, beneath, below—less than*
	Examples:	sublingual (sub-ling-gwal)—beneath the tongue subluxation (sub-luck-say-shun)—partial displacement of a bone from its joint (partial dislocation) submental (sub-men-tal)—beneath the chin (see meaning point)	
supra- (sue-prah)	Superman	Imagine Superman jumping over and above the Empire State building; is he high, or what?	*above, over, higher than, directly above*
	Examples:	supracostal (sue-prah-kos-tal)—above or outside the ribs supratentorial (sue-prah-ten-toh-ree-al)—above the tentorium of the cerebellum (therefore, above the brain) Some say "like over the head"	
syn- sym- (sin)	sin	Take away the breath of flowers; it would be a sin, and if you and I are not together, a sin times two. Is it a song or a thought?	*together*
	Examples:	syndactly (sin-dack-til-lee)—finger or digits together; the most common congenital defect affecting the hand symphysis (sim-fih-sis)—a type of joint in which the opposed bony surfaces are firmly united by a plate of fibrocartilage	

ELEMENT	MNEMONIC DEVICE	ASSOCIATION-IMAGE	MEANING
tarso- (tahr-sow)	torso	When you do this exercise, you bend at your mid-torso touching, your instep at the level of your ankle region. What is the exercise called?	[1]*ankle region, instep* [2]*framework of the upper eyelid*
	Examples:	tarsorrhaphy (tahr-sor-ah-fee)—the suturing of the upper and lower eyelids to shorten the opening of the eyelids tarsoclasis (tar-sok-lah-sis)—surgical fracturing of the tarsus of the foot	
tegument (teg-you-ment)	take a mint	When Joseph reached to take a mint, he noticed that the mint had a covering that looked just like pink skin; perhaps the mint was a little old! Yuk!	*skin or covering*
	Example:	integumentary (in-teg-you-men-tary) system; (sometimes called the common integument)—a term used to designate the entire covering of the body including not only the skin, but the other body coverings: hair; nails; and skin glands, including the mammary glands	
tens- (tenz)	tension	So much tension felt he, that it was as if his brain was being stretched into infinity; oh, the pain!	*stretch*
	Note:	The key to this element lies in the root ten- which carries a basic meaning of *stretch*, and is applied in medical terminology to convey the idea of *stretcher* or *stretching*. The root therefore appears in several forms:	
	Examples:	tendon (ten-don)—any of the cords of tough, fibrous connective tissue, which attach to muscle fibers and to bones, thereby causing motion by stretching and relaxing tenodesis (ten-odd-eh-sis)—suturing a tendon to bone tension (ten-shun)—the quality of being stretched or strained, or under pressure (psychotension?)	

ELEMENT	MNEMONIC DEVICE	ASSOCIATION-IMAGE	MEANING
thalam- (thal-am)	Thelma	Thelma, the fortune teller, had an inner chamber in her house where she would invite those who wished to have their fortunes told.	*inner chamber, gray mass located below the cerebrum*
	Examples:	thalamus (thal-ah-mus)—is located below the cerebrum thalamic (thal-ah-mick)—pertaining to the thalamus	
thel- (thel)	the L	In Jed's visual hallucination of the alphabet the L had a nipple for a top; wonder what Freud would say about that?	*nipple—a thin layer of tissue*
	Examples:	thelarche (the-lar-kee)—beginning of development of the breast at puberty epithelium (ep-ih-thee-lee-um)—specialized form of epithelial tissue that covers the external surfaces of the body as an outer layer of skin	
therap- (ther-ap)	the rap	The therapist stated, "I'll not take the rap because the word therapist is really two words, the and rapist; I was only doing my job." The judge did not agree.	*therapy*
	Example:	therapeutics (ther-ah-pew-ticks)—the science and art of healing; often the science is practiced without the warmth of the art	
therm- (therm) -thermia	thermos	A thermos is used to keep the heat in something, like coffee or tea.	*heat*
	Examples:	hyperthermia (hi-purr-ther-mee-ah)—an abnormally high body temperature; fever thermography (ther-mog-rah-fee)—technique using an infrared camera to photographically portray the body's surface temperature	

ELEMENT	MNEMONIC DEVICE	ASSOCIATION-IMAGE	MEANING
thorac- thoraco- (thoh-rah-koh)	Thor's act	It was Thor's act of throwing his hammer and it striking his opponent in the chest that ended the battle.	*chest*
	Examples:	thoracocentesis (thoh-ra-koh-sen-tee-sis)—puncture of the chest wall with a needle to obtain fluid from the pleural cavity thoracostomy (thoh-rah-kos-toh-me)—the surgical creation of a mouth or opening into the chest wall	
thrombo- (throm-boh)	throb	John's heartthrob brings a lump to his throat and a mucous clot to his nose; maybe it is just an allergy?	*lump, clot;* *coagulation*
	Examples:	thrombus (throm-bus)—a clot within a blood vessel thrombocytopenia (throm-boh-sigh-toh-pee-nee-ah)—abnormal decrease in the number of platelets	
-tope (tope)	tote	Jim was getting tired of having to tote all of his things from place to place; it was time to settle down.	*place, location*
	Examples:	ectopic (eck-top-ick)—situated elsewhere than in the normal place topical (top-ick-al)—pertaining to a particular location, as in topical anesthesia versus general anesthesia	
trachel- (tray-kel)	trickle	A small trickle of blood ran down her neckline; had she been bitten by a vampire, or had a love-bite gone wild?	*neck or neck-* *like structure*
	Examples:	trachea (tray-kee-ah)—name for the windpipe trachelocystitis (tray-kel-oh-sis-tye-tis)—inflammation of the neck of the bladder	
	Note:	The elements trache- and trachel- have different meanings, but closely resemble each other	

ELEMENT	MNEMONIC DEVICE	ASSOCIATION-IMAGE	MEANING
trans- (trans)	trance	When George was in a trance, it appeared that he looked across the room, through you and beyond and into infinity; only then was he able to communicate with the beyond.	*through, across, beyond*
	Examples:	transdermic (trans-derm-ick)—through the skin transplant (trans-plant)—planting across, as in skin grafting transnormal (trans-norm-al)—beyond normal, more than normal	
traumat- (traw-mat)	throw mat	"Throw mat," she said, "Don't you mean that old throw rug that looks like its been to war with all its injuries and wounds? It should be given a decent burial."	*wound, injury —shock stress*
	Examples:	traumatic (traw-mat-tick)—pertaining to trauma psychic trauma (traw-mah)—an emotional shock that makes a lasting impression on the mind, especially the subconscious mind	
trich- (trick)	trick	"My most famous trick," the magician said, "is growing hair on a golf ball."	*hair*
	Examples:	sclerotrichia (skler-oh-trick-ee-ah)—hard, dry state of hair trichoesthesia (trick-oh-es-thee-zee-ah)—"hair feeling" the sense by which one perceives that the hair of the skin is being touched	
trip- (trip) -tripsia	tripe	Jeb's statements were often tripe, rubbing people the wrong way, causing friction between them.	*rub, friction, crushing*
	Examples:	lithotripsy (lith-oh-trip-see)—crushing of a calculus (stone) within the kidney by the use of ultrasonic waves traveling through water tripsis (trip-sis)—the act of rubbing, massaging, or crushing	

ELEMENT	MNEMONIC DEVICE	ASSOCIATION-IMAGE	MEANING
-trophy (troh-fee)	trophy	One who has many a trophy can be said to demonstrate growth and development in his chosen sport.	*development, growth nutrition, nourishment*
	Examples:	atrophy (at-roh-fee)—weakness and wasting caused by disuse of the muscle over a long period (what you don't use, you lose) hypertrophy (high-per-troh-fee)—over development, the overgrowth of an organ or part	
tumor (tu-mor)	two more	If we keep adding two more of anything to something, I'm told that a swelling of everything will occur.	*swelling or enlargement*
	Note:	This word has been covered in the discussions of -oma and -onco; it is only put in here to provide you with a way of remembering that *tumor* means "swelling"	
turbin- (ter-bin)	turban	The great Horacio had a turban that was shaped like a top; perhaps if you pull one end; he will spin like a top.	*shaped like a top spiral-shaped*
	Examples:	turbinate (tur-bin-ate)—concha nasalis ossea turbinectomy (tur-bi-neck-toh-me)—excision of a nasal concha	
tympan- (tim-pan)	Tin Man	In my story the Tin Man is searching for an eardrum so that he can better hear the truth in the world.	*eardrum or its enclosure*
	Examples:	tympanic (tim-pan-ick)—pertaining to the eardrum tympanocentesis (tim-pah-no-sen-tee-sis)—surgical puncture of the tympanic membrane to remove fluid; also called myringotomy (mir-in-got-oh-me)	
umbilic- (um-bil-ick)	come Bill quick	Come Bill quick, look at the naval officer's parade; they are all wearing dress whites.	*navel—belly button*
	Example:	umbilical cord (um-bil-ih-kal kord)—the structure that connects the fetus to the placenta	

ELEMENT	MNEMONIC DEVICE	ASSOCIATION-IMAGE	MEANING
vaso- (vas-oh)	basso	Jim, a basso in the choir, could sing very low, so low that only a vessel in his neck gave clue to the fact that sound was being emitted.	*vessel*
	Examples:	vasoconstrictor (vas-oh-kon-strick-tor)—a drug that constricts (narrows) the blood vessels vasoneuropathy (vas-oh-new-rop-ah-thee)—a condition caused by combined vascular and neurologic defect, resulting from simultaneous action or interaction of the vascular and the nervous systems	
ventr- (ven-ter)	venture	"In this venture I want the money up front," he stated, "or we go belly up!"	*front, belly, abdomen*
	Examples:	ventral (ven-tral)—refers to the front or belly side of the body ventroptosis (ven-trop-toe-sis)—gastroptosis ventrocystorrhaphy (ven-troh-sist-or-ah-fee)—suturing of a cyst, or the bladder, to the abdominal wall	
vert- vers-) (vert)	pervert	Joey was hurt by Joan's words; just because he was reading PlayBoy magazine it didn't mean that he had turned into a pervert. Their relationship had just taken a turn for the worse.	*to turn, a turn*
	Examples:	vertebra (ver-teh-bra)—any of the single bones or segments of the spinal column that allow us to turn or twist our bodies retroversion (reh-troh-ver-shun)—the tipping backward of an entire organ vertigo (ver-tih-go)—a sense of whirling, dizziness, and the loss of balance	
vesic- (ves-ick)	Vlasic	Dawn held up a Vlasic pickle shaped like a urinary bladder, now the question was, how concrete was she—would she dare to eat it?	*bladder - urinary bladder also: blister*

ELEMENT	MNEMONIC DEVICE	ASSOCIATION-IMAGE	MEANING
	Examples:	vesicocele (ves-ick-koh-seel)—hernia of the bladder vesicant (ves-ih-kant)—producing blisters vesicle (ves-ih-kul)—circumscribed collection of clear fluid, also know as a blister	
vestibule (ves-tih-bule)	vestibule	A vestibule may be an entrance hall into a building or room.	*entrance—a space or cavity at the entrance to a canal*
	Examples:	vestibulogenic (vs-tib-you-loh-jen-ick)—arising in a vestibule, as that of the ear labial vestibule (lay-bee-al ves-tih-bule)—that portion of the vestibule of the mouth which lies between the lips, and the teeth and gums	
viscero- (vis-er-oh)	vicious	The organ grinder had a monkey that was vicious and would bite you if you came too close.	*organ—an internal organ*
	Examples:	visceral (vis-er-al)—pertaining to an internal organ, especially those of the abdomen viscerad (vis-er-ad)—toward the viscera visceroptosis (vis-er-op-toe-sis)—a dropping or falling down of the viscera; for example, due to weakness in the abdominal muscles—gravity will have its way with you	
-vulse (vul-se)	pulse	It is difficult to take the radial pulse of someone with a nervous twitch as they may pull away involuntarily.	*twitch or pull - pluck tear loose*
	Examples:	avulsion (ah-vul-shun)—the tearing away of a structure or part as in an avulsion fracture convulsion (kon-vul-shun)—a pulling together; involuntary spasm or contraction of muscles	

CHAPTER ELEVEN

ELEMENT APPERCEPTION EXERCISE

Pronounce the word aloud, and then break down the word into its elements. Define the elements by stating the meaning of the last element first, then the other elements in that same order.

Example: Word = Encephalorrhexis = a breaking, a bursting or rupture; the head and within, or the brain; therefore the meaning might be: to blow one's mind.

1.	sublingual	20.	subluxation
2.	supracostal	21.	supratentorial
3.	syndactly	22.	symphysis
4.	tarsorrhaphy	23.	tarsoclasis
5.	common integument	24.	tenodesis
6.	thalamus	25.	thelarche
7.	epithelium	26.	therapeutics
8.	hyperthermia	27.	thermography
9.	thoracocentesis	28.	thoracostomy
10.	thrombocytopenia	29.	ectopic
11.	trachelocystitis	30.	transdermic
12.	tramatologist	31.	sclerotrichia
13.	trichoesthesia	32.	lithotripsy
14.	hypertrophy	33.	atrophy
15.	tumorigenesis	34.	turbinectomy
16.	tympanocentesis	35.	umbilical
17.	vasoneuropathy	36.	ventrocystorrhaphy
18.	retroversion	37.	vesicocele
19.	vestibulogenic	38.	viscerad

MEANING POINT

Schizophrenia [Gr. schizein, to split; phren, mind] as a word does indeed mean "split mind." What the meaning should relate is that this is a brain disease that causes one to be split from reality in some way. As a diagnosis, Schizophrenia presents with delusions (false beliefs), prominent hallucinations (voices in one's head that no one else can hear, or visual images that no other can see), incoherence, or marked loosening of associations (loss of logical, connected thinking where one thought may not connect with another), catatonic behavior (lead pipe flexibility, where one can stand for hours without moving while allowing extremities to be moved, after which they will remain where moved), flat or grossly inappropriate affect (no expression at all, or a smile while telling one that their mother died). Often the foregoing is referred to as a psychotic process, and, therefore, Schizophrenia is considered a psychosis rather than a neurosis.

Mental—This may be either of two terms, each having a different derivation. (1) Latin—*mens, mentia,* the mind. Thus mental, referring to the mind. (2) Latin—*mentum,* the chin. Thus mental, referring to the chin.

In this section of the test you will find a short story made up of the *association-images* found in your book. There are 10. Not all paragraphs will contain an *association-image* that refer to a medical word element, some will contain more than one. Minor changes in grammatical syntax have been made to the *association-images* to tell the story. At the end of the story put down in the appropriate paragraph number the word, or words, that you believe have been indicated. Remember, the words you write are medical word elements, not lay terms. As an example in the following sentence: The card is the ace of hearts. You would put down the medical element card—or cardio-, not the word heart. *Please* put only the word(s) refered to in the correct paragraph number. If the paragraph number does not match the correct medical element, it may be counted as a wrong answer.

NIGHT FISHIN'

1. It wuz a Saturday night 'bout midnight when John comes in fer a pint er two, draggin' a wee wet rag of a man behind him. "What's dooin'?" sez I, tryin' not ta laugh at th' manikin, who I recognizes at once.

2. "Ye'll ne'er believe it," sez he. "I wuz strollin' along the docks fer a bit o' fresh air, when I smells th' most awful stench. Th' rancid odor seeped through, as if by osmosis, th' wet cloth I held ta me nose, but I proceeded anyway. I follows me nose, an' what do I see but this wee bit of a man, shiverin' an' shakin', all wet an' blue with th' cold, just swimmin' up ta th' shore. The patchy fog wuz so darned thick he couldna spy th' land, and he swims right up onta th' shingle!"

3. "Yer a liar," sez Joe. "Them waters is full o' sharks that'll eat a man up afore he can swim two strokes!" Joe's raffish comment caused him pain and the need fer eight sutures, 'cause our Johnny's not th' type o' man ta take an insult like that. Up he jumps, bearin' down on puir Joe like a bald Irish Fury, when Wham! In his scurry, John trips and falls hard on his posterior—oh the pain!—and misses puir Joe entirely.

4. As fer the wee wet man, his posture needed adjustment since his back part was protrudin', and it was this that caused Johnny ta miss. Instead, he smacks into the wet man, who knocks his skull into Joe's lip, splittin' it open. At this the wee man lets out a yelp as would shame a banshee, and darts outta th' door.

5. Now, I know Johny's tellin' th' truth. When John tells a fib, I can always tell 'cause he has a large vein in his neck that stands out, and I canna see it atall. Afore I can get this across ta puir Joe, bleedin' all inta his beer, the wee wet man comes back

w' th' coppers, yammerin' about how he wuz kidnapped an' then assaulted by our Johnny, beggin' ta have Johnny arested, and threatnin' ta sue him ta boot.

6. Th' Inspector sez, "A foe may be one to fear, if such a man is here, but this crime is quite ridiculous, we'll have to get to the root of it soon." So Johnny starts tellin' him about the wee man an' the smell an' the docks an' the swim, an' th' Inspector ain't buyin' it nohow. He cuffs Johnny and heads fer th' door, with him yellin' out loud a they hauls him away, "I'm bein' sued under false pretenses, I tell ya!"

7. After it quiets down a bit, an' Joe gets off ta be swn up, I'm sittin' w' a fresh pint in me hand, shakin' me head an' mutterin' under me breath, "puir Johnny, fer once he tells th' truth an' still gets hauled away!"

8. "What makes ye think it were th' truth he wuz tellin'?" sez Paddy, th' barkeep.

9. "Well ye see, I knows who that wee wet man is all about bein'," sez I, not wantin' ta give away th' secret about the vein in Johnny's neck. "He's a solicitor fer those as has been in accidents an' th' like. Me brother-in-law which is a patrolman tells me th' sorry little runt shows up at wrecks on th' highway afore th' ambulance most times. Sez it reminds him o' how th' sharks show up when he chums th' water off his fishin' boat."

10. "I don't see how that means that Johnny wusna tellin' a lie," sez Paddy.

11. "Easy," sez I. "Like Joe sez, there's sharks thick as Johnny's skull in them waters, and as ye well know, those who believe it's true that a shark may eat the flesh of its own kind are wrong. Shark is about th' only thing another shark willna eat; an' it's by their singular stench they recognizes each other. Of course th' wee man wusna bothered by em'—'tis only professional courtesy!"

ANSWERS

1. _____
2. _____
3. _____
4. _____
5. _____
6. _____
7. _____
8. _____
9. _____
10. _____
11. _____

In this section of the test you will find a short story made up of the *association-images* found in your book. There are 10. All paragraphs will contain an *association-image* that refer to a medical word element. At the end of the story put down in the appropriate paragraph number the word that you believe has been indicated. Remember, these words you write are medical word elements, not lay terms. As an example in the following sentence: The card in the ace of hearts. You would put down the medical element card—or cardio-, not the word heart.

A GATHERING OF MINDS

1. Rudy was the first to enter the group setting. Rudy had several complexes with an interweaving network of anxieties that abraded his conscious reality to the point of madness, at times.

2. Next Patty came and sat in her usual chair facing the window. It was said that Patty had a flat affect; I thought concave to be more descriptive.

3. John was the third to enter and he started the group with the comment, "Some say I am free because I can move around on both sides of my internal world of mind, left and right, as if in two ways of thinking."

4. John went on to say that, his mind was in mint condition; but, I'm not so sure that is a positive statement these days.

5. Patty took out a facial tissue. She had a history of allergic coryza with much use of facial tissue to blow her nose.

6. Then John blurted out, "History has told us of great womb-mates by one who utters to us hysterically; could this be true?" he went on.

7. I thought it time that I directed the conversation and said, "If one experiences an up and down cycle of mood swings it may be that he has a bipolar mind, called manic depressive psychosis—or illness. Is that what you are referring to John?"

8. John answered, "A feeling of ecstasy may cause one to inspire to full expansion one's lungs—but not necessarily be manic; besides I take my lithium Doc."

9. Rudy interrupted, "Some say that lithium is a stone in the armamentarium of psychiatry, it sounds archaic to me, and perhaps they pushed the metaphor too far!"

10. Patty turned away from the window to face the group, held out her hand and said, "If you listen, you can hear both voice and sound coming from my disconnected phone," as if there was a phone in her hand. Then added, "Perhaps it's only my voices, Doc."

11. It was about time for the group to be over. Although it often didn't seem like we accomplished a great deal during group, I knew deep inside that this was not necessarily true. There are those who would make small of a group such as this, but they may be a bit shortsighted. Sometime all that is needed is contact with another person to prevent aloneness from engulfing reality. For but for the grace of God, there go I. For these few souls, in this sick system of mental health that is falling, even this brief verbal touch may cement sanity together for yet another day. Tomorrow however, is still yet to come.

ANSWERS

1. _____
2. _____
3. _____
4. _____
5. _____
6. _____
7. _____
8. _____
9. _____
10. _____
11. _____

In this section of the test you will find a short story made up of the *association-images* found in your book. There are 10. Not all paragraphs will contain an *association-image* that refer to a medical word element. Some paragraphs will have more than one. Minor changes in grammatical syntax have been made to the *association-images* to tell the story. At the end of the story put down in the appropriate paragraph number the word(s) that you believe have been indicated. Remember, these words you write are medical word elements, not lay terms.

THE CIRCUS

1. When the circus comes to town, it seems like everyone becomes a kid again. Everyone loves to go to the circus. Often the first person you will see is the clown.

2. The clown was giving out free cotton candy in front of the circus tent before anyone had a chance to buy it inside.

3. The clown had a parrot named Polly, he said, "My parrot Polly has many bright colors, she's too much!" Then we started to laugh when Polly said, "He's a friend of mine." Everyone was surprised to hear Polly say that, it came out so clear.

4. Thelma, the fortuneteller, had an inner chamber in her tent where she would invite those who wished to have their fortune told. But, this was not Thelma's only job, she also sang in the inner ring.

5. The clown came to Thelma's tent and told her it was time for her to go to the Main tent to sing her song, she had to sing her song at the top of the spiral staircase in the inner ring in the Main tent. So off she went to the Main tent and climbed the spiral staircase. When she reached the top of the spiral staircase, she looked down at the coil of stairs below and became quite dizzy. But, after a few seconds, she was ready to sing.

6. Then at the sideshow, the great Horacio (the magician) was doing his magic tricks. "My most famous trick," the magician said, "Is growing hair on a golf ball." The great Horacio had a turban shaped like a top; perhaps if you pull one end he will spin like a top.

7. The organ grinder had a monkey that was vicious and would bite if you came to close. The children did not get close to the organ grinder; instead, they went to see the balloon man. He had many balloons.

8. Wouldn't it be something if balloons could talk. For instance, one balloon to another, "What really wrecks us is one tiny pin, it causes us to break or burst."

9. The children continued playing games on the midway. The plastic balls being blown in the air by jets of air fascinated them. In fact, they caught a few. The man who ran the game said, "If one puts a hole in a plastic ball one must then do some plastic repair." The children said they would not put any holes in the plastic balls. Finally, it was time to go home, sleepy and tired, but oh what fun!!

10. Then, when the circus leaves town, everyone goes back to their normal lives, and they wait until next year when the circus comes back again.

ANSWERS

1. _____
2. _____
3. _____
4. _____
5. _____
6. _____
7. _____
8. _____
9. _____
10. _____
11. _____

CHAPTER TWELVE

MNEMONICS

ELEMENT	MNEMONIC DEVICE	ASSOCIATION-IMAGE	MEANING
adip(o)- (ad-ih-po)	dip stick	Visualize the mechanic pulling your oil dip stick; then—it begins to grow very fat.	*fat*
	Example:	adipoid (ad-ih-poid)—lipoid	
-ary (airy)	airy	When Joe puts on an airy way, it pertains to his internal thinking; thinking that tells him, he is better than others—poor sap!	*pertains to*
	Example:	urinary (you-rih-nary)—pertaining to urine	
aort(o)- (ay-or-toe)	oratory	Jim made great claims during his oratory debut, claiming that he could constrict one's aorta by mere thought, a process of psychokinesis.	*aorta*
	Example:	aortic (ay-or-tick)—pertaining to the aorta	
ather(o)- (ath-er-oh)	rather	Rather than being thought of as a fat, ugly boy with plaque on his teeth, Dan took to weight lifting and brushing his teeth.	*plaque, fatty*
	Example:	atherosclerosis (ath-er-oh-skleh-roh-sis)—hardening and narrowing of the arteries due to a buildup of cholestrol plaques	

ELEMENT	MNEMONIC DEVICE	ASSOCIATION-IMAGE	MEANING
cutane(o)- (kyou-tay-no)	curtain	Jerry pulled the thin curtain over act three of the play. The curtain was so thin, that it appeared to be a fine skin separating the audience from the stage play; an eerie effect indeed!	*skin*
	Example:	cutaneous (kyou-tay-nee-us)—pertaining to the skin	
lute(o)- (lue-tee-oh)	flute	Rudy was to play a yellow flute made of bamboo. Evidently, they did not have a shiny metal one.	*yellow or the corpus luteum*
	Example:	lutein (lue-tee-in)—a pigment found in nature from latin *luteus* = yellow	
-necrosis (neh-kroh-sis)	neck roses	Jody wore neck roses of garlic to hide the death of tissue she had due to leprosy; or was it to fend off further attacks from the village vampire?	*death of tissue*
	Example:	arterionecrosis (ar-tee-ree-oh-neh-kroh-sis)—means death of an artery or arteries	
nulli- (nuh-lee)	null	Christopher made no attempt to respond to the question; it was a question filled with the null of contempt and the best answer was none.	*none*
	Example:	nulligravida (null-ih-grav-ih-dah)—a woman who has never been pregnant	
olig(o)- (ol-ih-goh)	ogled	There were scanty few eyes that ogled Catherine after the age of 45, a fact that began to affect her work since she was a movie star. Were the days of glamour gone forever?	*scanty, few*

ELEMENT	MNEMONIC DEVICE	ASSOCIATION-IMAGE	MEANING
	Example:	oligophrenia (ol-ih-goh-free-nee-ah)—mental deficiency	
pharyng(o)- (far-ing-goh)	flamingo	Carol had a flamingo with bright red coloring about its throat.	*pharynx - throat*
	Example:	pharyngorrhagia (far-ing-goh-ray-jee-ah)—bleeding from the pharynx	
primi- (prye-mi)	prime	During school, it seemed as if Carl wanted prime time with his teacher because he was always first in line when the teacher asked for volunteers.	*first*
	Example:	primipara (prye-mip-ah-rah)—woman who has borne one child	
-rrhea (ree-ah)	Korea	Rufus got his military discharge while in Korea.	*to flow, discharge*
	Example:	urethrorrhea (you-ree-throh-ree-ah)—abnormal discharge from the urethra	
ureter(o) urethra -uria ur/o		All four pertain to the urinary system.	*ureter* *urethra* *urination, urine urine, urinary tract*

CHAPTER TWELVE

ELEMENT APPERCEPTION EXERCISE

Pronounce the word aloud, and then break down the word into its elements. Define the elements by stating the meaning of the last element first, then the other elements in the same order.

Example: Word = olighypomenorrhea = flow, menses, scanty or infrequent menstruation with diminished menstral flow.

1.	adipoid	11.	urinary
2.	aortic stenosis	12.	cutaneous
3.	lutein	13.	arterionecrosis
4.	nulligravida	14.	oligophrenia
5.	pharyngorrhagia	15.	primipara
6.	urocele	16.	luteinization
7.	adiposuria	17.	oligoencephalon
8.	diarrhea	18.	atherosclerosis
9.	asepticnecrosis	19.	osteonecrosis
10.	axillary	20.	oligodontia

MEANING POINT:

Axilla (Latin-armpit) The derivation is uncertain. It has been suggested that it is a compound word formed from *axis alae*, meaning axle of the wing, because the arm or wing revolves from this point. It is also suggested that it is diminutive of *ala*, wing, since a number of Latin terms have undergone similiar change, e.g. *mala*, cheek, from maxilla; *talus*, an anklebone, from taxillus; *tela*, a web, from texilla; etc. There is also a late Latin form *ascella*. In English, as axilla since 1600.

FINAL EXAMINATION
MEDICAL TERMINOLOGY

acousti-	_____	acro-	_____
aer-	_____	ambi-	_____
an-, a-	_____	anti-	_____
-asthenia	_____	auto-	_____
blephar-	_____	carcin-	_____
caust-	_____	celio-	_____
cervic-	_____	chondr-	_____
colla-	_____	cor	_____
crani-	_____	-crine	_____
cyan-	_____	dacry-	_____
dendr-	_____	-desis	_____
dura	_____	-ectasis	_____
-ectomy	_____	encephal-	_____
ependym-	_____	fascia	_____
furca-	_____	gemin-	_____
gingiv-	_____	gluco-	_____
gravid	_____	hallux-	_____
hepat-	_____	histo-	_____
hypo-	_____	-iasis	_____
intra-	_____	kerat-	_____
lacrim-	_____	leuk-	_____
lith-	_____	lumbo-	_____
macul-	_____	malign-	_____

maxill-	_____	melan-	_____
metabol(e)	_____	myco-	_____
nephr-	_____	olfact-	_____
oment-	_____	onych-	_____
ophthalm-	_____	orth-	_____
orchi-	_____	-ostomy	_____
pachy-	_____	pariet-	_____
peps-	_____	phak-	_____
phleb-	_____	phrag-	_____
-plegia	_____	pod-	_____
poster-	_____	proct-	_____
pseud-	_____	pyloro-	_____
radi-	_____	radic-	_____
ramus	_____	retr(o)-	_____
salpingo-	_____	scirr(h)-	_____
semen	_____	somato-	_____
spiro-	_____	squam-	_____
strept-	_____	supra-	_____
tegument	_____	thel-	_____
-tope	_____	trich-	_____
tumor	_____	vaso-	_____
vesic-	_____	viscero-	_____

SECTION II
STORY FORMAT

In this section of the final, you will find a short story made up of the *association-images* found in your book. There are 10 word elements to be found. Not all paragraphs will contain an *association-image* that refers to a medical word element. Some will have 2. However, there are 10. At the end of the story put down in the appropriate paragraph number the word(s) that you believe have been indicated. Remember, these are medical word elements, not lay terms. These are not bonus questions. Minor changes in grammatical syntax have been made to the *association-images* to tell the story—however, all element references remain intact and can be easily identified.

THE CASE OF THE LATENT FILM

1. Joe Spade sat in his office. Business was slow, bills were unpaid; but, there was always the next moment.

2. The door opened to his PI office and a buxom blonde came in. Joe thought to himself, astronomy is the study of the heavenly bodies, some of which are star shaped; and she was no exception, of coarse, she wasn't star shaped, perhaps just a star.

3. Jane was her name. Her problem, the missing film—film that told a tale.

4. "In this venture I want the money up front," Joe said, "or we go belly up!"

5. Jane came across with his fee and then left.

6. Joe left his office, he had one clue, but first he had to talk with inspector Justin Jowls.

7. Joe entered the inspector's office. After a few moments of talking with the inspector, the inspector said, "This crime is quite ridiculous; we'll have to get to the root of it soon!"

8. Joe next went to his church, a place where he used to go with his girlfriend Virginia. Sitting on the cold pew, he was at once aware of the hollow space beside him where Virginia used to sit.

9. A man came into the church and sat next to Joe. He whispered that he knew of the latent film. Joe said, "You are nothing but a windbag, Sir, full of hot air."

Then, the man threw a fist at Joe's jaw. Joe ducked, escaping within a narrow margin the full force of the blow that may have given him an early passage to bedtime. Joe returned the blow with devastating results and the man left running out of the church.

10. As Joe gave chase, another man, sitting near by, grabbed Joe by the arm asking him why he was chasing the man who left. Joe's raffish comment caused him pain and the need for eight sutures.

11. Back at his office Joe sat nursing his sore jaw. Jane came in. Joe thought, I smell a rodent here. It is a known old fact that smell brings about the most primitive recall—and response. Joe grabbed Jane by the arm and said, "There are ways to loosen your tongue, so don't lie sis." Poor technique for a PI, don't you think?

12. Then Joe spied a film out of the corner of his eye, a roll of film not yet developed, unseen by any eyes, latent and waiting.

13. The film was there all the time. Jane had left it on his couch—maybe on purpose; but, it didn't make any difference now, the case was solved.

ANSWERS

1. _____
2. _____
3. _____
4. _____
5. _____
6. _____
7. _____
8. _____
9. _____
10. _____
11. _____

FINAL EXAMINATION—2
MEDICAL TERMINOLOGY

acousti-	_____	aden-	_____
adnexa-	_____	aveol-	_____
ambi-	_____	ameb-	_____
angi-	_____	ante-	_____
antr-	_____	arthr-	_____
-asthenia	_____	aur-	_____
benign	_____	cata-	_____
-centesis	_____	cephal-	_____
cheir-	_____	-clasis	_____
dactyl-	_____	dendr-	_____
-desis	_____	dors-	_____
dura	_____	-ectasis	_____
-ectomy	_____	encephal-	_____
ependym-	_____	-esthesia	_____
eu-	_____	fascia	_____
gangli-	_____	geron-	_____
gingiv-	_____	glosso-	_____
glyco-	_____	hallux	_____
hepat-	_____	hydro-	_____
hyster-	_____	infra-	_____
iso-	_____	kerat-	_____
lacrim-	_____	later-	_____

lingua	_____	lith-	_____
macul-	_____	malign-	_____
maxill-	_____	mening-	_____
metabol(e)	_____	myco-	_____
myring-	_____	ocul-	_____
olfact-	_____	onych-	_____
ortho-	_____	orchi-	_____
osmo-	_____	oto-	_____
pachy-	_____	para-	_____
path-	_____	-penia	_____
phob-	_____	phragma-	_____
phren-	_____	platy-	_____
-plegia	_____	pneum-	_____
-podia	_____	proct-	_____
-ptosis	_____	pyloro-	_____
rhin-	_____	salpingo-	_____
-scopy	_____	sedat-	_____
somni-	_____	spondyl-	_____
stoma-	_____	supra-	_____
thalam-	_____	thrombo-	_____
-tripsia	_____	turbin-	_____
tympan-	_____	ventr-	_____
vesic-	_____	viscero-	_____

FINAL EXAMINATION
PART TWO
STORY FORMAT (10 QUESTIONS)

In this section of the test you will find a short story made up of the *association-images* found in your book. There are 10, one in each paragraph. Minor changes in grammatical syntax have been made to the *association-images* to tell the story—however, all element references remain intact and can be easily identified. At the end of the story put down in the appropriate paragraph number the word that you believe has been indicated. Remember, these words you write are medical word elements, not lay terms. *Example:* When the reference is to heart put down the element cardi-; in this case, the mnemonic device is card, as in the ace of hearts.

A CLIMB TO FAME

1. When Jane first met Joe he was a most dynamic speaker; his power to control an audience was something to see.

2. How well Jane remembered that first time Joe was speaking when he said, "May the devil's fire cause you to burn eternally," but he was only reading a line from a play.

3. Joe was lecturing an audience of young teaching students. "When unsure of his rhetoric a teacher may take a step backwards while lecturing," he said in a knowing tone.

4. Joe continued, "As a writer some say I am free because I can move around on both sides of my internal world of mind, left and right, as if in two ways of thinking. Poetry may allow us to exist in many ways of thinking.

5. Evidently this statement was a lead to Joe's new book on poetry because his next statement was, "A prologue to my book is a poem in front of the book that you read before you actually start reading the book, I hope!"

6. Joe quoted a brief line from his book, "Be mine, mild or hot, for only love, not love me not, can serve us both."

7. Joe went on to talk about art and poetry, next reading a perfume bottle label that read, "Kiss me Quick!" and depicted two large red lips pursed as if to entice one to kiss without restrain.

8. That was Joe's beginning, his life of fame was grasped in gradual steps, taken ad lib, without the passion of love, but with the cool calm of deliberation; what a pity.

9. Joe's eventual fame was to be tarnished by one of his fears. Although an able combat veteran, Joe could not get far enough away from spiders, it was a real phobia, arachnophobia.

10. But even his fear pushed him on to greater fame and he wrote his first best seller with the title, "A foe may be one to fear, but a phobia can be from there to here."

11. But, that was many years and books ago. Fame has long since had its way with him, and now he resides only in our mind's eye; God bless you Joe, we love you yet.

ANSWERS

1. _____
2. _____
3. _____
4. _____
5. _____
6. _____
7. _____
8. _____
9. _____
10. _____
11. _____

NOTES:

MEDICAL TERMINOLOGY
FINAL EXAM 3

acousti-	_____	erythro-	_____
adnexa-	_____	-esthesia	_____
alveol-	_____	eu-	_____
ameb-	_____	fascia	_____
amphi-	_____	furca-	_____
-asthenia	_____	geron-	_____
auto-	_____	gingiv-	_____
blephar-	_____	glosso-	_____
cantho-	_____	hallux	_____
capit-	_____	heter-	_____
cata-	_____	hydro-	_____
caus-	_____	hypno-	_____
cec-	_____	hyster-	_____
-centesis	_____	infra-	_____
cerebr-	_____	iso-	_____
cheil-	_____	kerat-	_____
chondr-	_____	lal-	_____
colla-	_____	leio-	_____
cyan-	_____	lingua	_____

dacry-	_____	lith-	_____
dactyl-	_____	-malacia	_____
duct-	_____	malign-	_____
-ectasis	_____	melan-	_____
encephal-	_____	myo-	_____
myring-	_____		
ocul-	_____		

odont-	_____	salpingo-	_____
olfact-	_____	schizo-	_____
-oma	_____	sclera-	_____
onych-	_____	semen	_____
ortho-	_____	somni-	_____
osmo-	_____	sphenic	_____
oto-	_____	strepto-	_____
palpebra-	_____	syn-	_____
part-	_____	tegument	_____
-penia	_____	thalam-	_____
-pexy	_____	thel-	_____
phak-	_____	thrombo-	_____
phob-	_____	trans-	_____

phrax- _____

plak- _____

-plasty _____

-plegia _____

-podia _____

poster- _____

pro- _____

psued- _____

ptyal- _____

ramus _____

-rrhexis _____

-trophy _____

ventr- _____

viscero- _____

FINAL EXAMINATION STORY TEST

In this section of the final exam you will find a short story made up of the association | images found in your book. There are ten (10) word elements to be identified. Not all paragraphs will contain an association | image that refer to a medical word element. Some paragraph(s) may have two. However, there are ten to be found. There have been minor changes in wording to correct for grammar, otherwise the association | image(s) remain intact and should be identifiable. At the end of the story put down across from the appropriate paragraph number the medical word element(s) that you believe have been indicated. Remember, these are medical word elements not lay terms representing medical elements. As in cardi—for heart.

THE ARGUMENT

1. It has been said that a good argument often clears the air for the better, I wonder? The following may prove different—please read on.

2. Jake and Joe were often friends, sometimes opponents, always in disagreement about something. And for the record, It is a well-known fact, if you interfere with an argument between two people, you may be among the injured. Today their friends gave no heed to this aphorism.

3. In any discussion, Jeb's statements were often tripe, rubbing people the wrong way causing friction between them. Today was such a day. Joe and Jake were having a heated discussion regarding capital punishment. Joe had stated that he was against the death penalty. Jake had naturally taken the opposite stand—and with good reason, he had pointed out, "You don't have to feed the dead."

4. "Your mind is a great void, resembling the vastness of outer space," Jake said, looking Joe directly in the eyes, glaring. Joe replied, "And yours liken to a vacuum it would seem; what keeps your ears from collapsing upon themselves?"

5. Kyle, sitting nearby, chimed in, "He certainly seems to be a high person, maybe aloof is a better description, a more than normal pain in the posterior." Jeb noticed out loud, that an opinion was like an anus, everyone either was one, or had one, he couldn't remember which?

6. However, Joe's raffish comment caused him pain and the need for eight sutures as Jake had pasted him a good one over his left eye.

7. Kyle stood up when someone (Jake) had said, "Shut up," (now) he has a fat lip.

8. Jeb stated, "A foe may be one to fear, but he's a friend of mine—so he walked over and Jake gave him a punch in the mouth.

9. Jeb left hurriedly yelling over his shoulder, "You are nothing but a windbag, Sir, full of hot air." But he made sure that he was out of the building before he finished; he didn't need another punch in the eye.

10. So—three down, none to go. Jake felt bad. Joe was holding his handkerchief over his left eye. Joe looked at Jake. Jake looked back at Joe. They both started laughing, "Hell, that was a real doozie, look at this mess." Arm in arm they left for the emergency room. It was suture time. I guess they were real friends, but you can leave me out of the their friendship next time. Someone was saying, "It isn't any secret, crying over spilled milk is a waste of time!"

ANSWERS

1. _____
2. _____
3. _____
4. _____
5. _____
6. _____
7. _____
8. _____
9. _____
10. _____
11. _____

NOTES:

APPENDICES

PRACTICE IN STORY FORMAT

In this section you will find a short story made up of the association-images found in your lessons. There are 16 word elements to be found. Not all paragraphs will contain an association-image that refers to a medical word element. Some may have two. However, there are 16. At the end of the story, put down in the appropriate paragraph number the word(s) that you believe have been indicated. Remember, these are medical word elements that you will be putting down, not lay terms.

THE CASE OF THE AILING SCRIPT

1. Oliver P. Shagnasty's only claim to fame, it seemed, resided in his recently completed play. At forty he had put most of his eggs in one basket, that being this play with the title, "*Love Comes to Roost*," a three act play about Sir Hic the knight in shining armor, a girl that is the knight's friend, and the Tin Man; an unusual love triangle, to say the least.

2. The director and fabulous playwright, Howard Knowles, was being quite critical. He said, "The first act, to me, needs to be cut, in part or all, if this play is to survive."

3. The director was an impolite little man with beady eyes and no sense of humor. They said that his diplomatic protocol was not fit for man or beast, calling him an *anus equines*, or worse. It was that worse that Oliver uttered, words proclaiming something about Howard's parentage, and that started the argument.

4. Howard looked at Oliver and said that his posture needed adjustment since his back part was protruding; just the thing for a good kicking.

5. I decided it was time to break this up and get back to the business at hand, knowing that if you interfere with an argument between two people, you may be among the injured.

6.	After a few more words they were at a standstill; what I saw were two equal values in logic since they both agreed on at least one premise, and in a syllogistic way, this confirmed the outcome for me. Even a TV series bases one epic upon another, in addition to being continued *ad infinitum.* (ahd ihn-fee-NEE-tuum)

7.	However, it is the movement from one scene to another that creates a story during a movie; and your persistence of vision that creates image movement—for this play, persistence of thought would assist with understanding. It was time to get back to the play. I asked Oliver to read/discuss more of the script.

8.	"OK" he said, "Let's see, Sir Hic, a knight in shining armor often caught it in the neck while jousting." "Poor adjustment, I would say," I added with a sheepish grin.

9.	What came next in the play was a love scene. Oliver's favorite line was, "Be mine, mild or hot, for only love, not love me not, can serve us both."

10.	Ed Mayhem came in, late and drunk as usual, and made the comment quite loud, "We need a commercial here. Imagine a girl named Melanie; she's wearing black boots and saying," "These boots are made for walking." I interrupted, telling Ed to sit down and listen. Thinking to myself, drinking alcohol before any activity that requires critical thinking may be mulling to the mind, even harmful, producing bad outcomes in thinking.

11.	Oliver continued, "In my story, the Tin Man is searching for an eardrum so that he can better hear the truth in the world."

12.	At this time, Patricia Nelson, Oliver's girlfriend, interjected her point of view. "What about this line, Oliver?" She was way ahead of us in her reading of the script. She read: "John's heartthrob brings a lump to his throat and a mucous clot to his nose." "Maybe it's just an allergy," she said innocently. I thought to myself, her portrayal of pure innocence was childlike, but not necessarily vestal.

13.	At this point Ed jumped up and yelled, "It is said that Salvadore Dali painted a picture where toast is soggy, drooping and falling." Sounds like my breakfast, I thought to myself. Evidently Ed was trying to help, but what Ed said was against and counter to the present system of belief (for the play), and a contradiction in terms as well. We weren't doing a play in surrealism.

14.	Well, time has had its way with his play. Oliver never became known for it, but years later, after his death, he was known for a feature article he had written. Life is strange that way.

Write Your Answers Below

Paragraph   1   _____

Paragraph   2   _____

Paragraph   3   _____

Paragraph   4   _____

Paragraph   5   _____

Paragraph   6   _____

Paragraph   7   _____

Paragraph   8   _____

Paragraph   9   _____

Paragraph   10   _____

Paragraph   11   _____

Paragraph   12   _____

Paragraph   13   _____

Paragraph   14   _____

Remember, not all paragraphs have two words, and some do not have any word. Also remember, you are writing down the medical element, not the lay term. Example: *cardi-*, not heart. Example: "toast is" = ptosis when defining. Enjoy.

EXAMPLE OF TRANSCRIPTION

The following example is not taken from an actual recording, and the information does not relate to any real case history. The information is purely fictional. The subject matter is based on multiple real histories in many manuals, books, and information derived from the DSM-IV (Diagnostic and Statistical Manual of Mental Disorders, 4th Edition), to name only a few. The pathology demonstrated could be real. The situation depicted is fictional. However, as it exists, it gives a realistic representation of the pathology that could exist in such a case history.

IDENTIFYING DATA:

This is my initial contact with this 32-year-old caucasian female. She is approximately 5'5", buxom, blond, with a pallid complexion. She is dressed in appropriate attire for her age. She is admitted on a 5150 status for psychiatric observation due to an aberrant behavior pattern for the last seven days as well as possible danger to her infant son.

HISTORY OF PRESENT PROBLEM:

The patient came to the attention of her family because "she seemed to be different," according to her husband. After recently (about six weeks) giving birth to a nine-pound-five ounce boy, she began to say strange things and seemed depressed. Primary reason for this 1st admission has to do with the patient leaving her six-week-old infant alone in his crib and the patient being found in town in a bar trying to engage a male in a sexual liaison. Her reason, she stated: "God has made me the mother of all men. They are just little boys, you know!"

She has no previous mental health history and she is in good physical condition. Childbirth was normal. There are no known problems of childhood and she takes no drugs or alcohol, other than that which is prescribed by her family doctor. In fact, her being in the bar was quite unusual, according to her family, as she has never had a drinking problem or ever taken a drink, even on special occasions. She was often referred to by other family members as being a teetotaler.

MENTAL STATUS EXAM:

The patient presents as petite, immaculate in dress, with a strong odor of perfume and appropriate makeup. She comes to the interview willingly. She offers no complaint, but states, "I'm on a mission to save all men from their sexual fantasies." She offers no reason, other than the one given initially, for her behavior—in fact does not seem to be aware of the implications of what she has done, stating only that God has spoken to her. She denies suicidal thoughts and is without concommitant suicidal ideation otherwise. At times, there is a flight of ideas, and she attends to internal stimuli. She is basically oriented in time, person, and place. There is a grandiosity to her speech content that almost seems bipolar. There is no evidence of memory impairment, confusion, clouding of sensorium, or other signs of organic brain disease or schizophrenia.

DIAGNOSTIC IMPRESSION:

Axis I	298.90 Psychotic Disorder, NOS
	R/O Post Partum Psychosis
	R/O Bipolar Psychosis
Axis II	V71.09 None noted
Axis III	Post Partum X six weeks
Axis IV	Stressors 3—moderate (childbirth)
Axis V	Current: 25
	Highest: 80

TREATMENT PLAN:

1. Evaluation for medication after routine tests.
2. The patient will be involved in the general ward milieu.
3. The patient will be involved in individual and group psychotherapy while on the ward.
4. Close collaboration with the patient's family prior to release and an investigation and/or follow-up past history in more detail by social worker while patient is on the ward.

COMMONLY ACCEPTED ABBREVIATIONS
A FRACTIONAL LIST

ab	antibody
ABC	airway, breathing, circulation
a.c.	before meals
AC	assist control
ACh	acetylcholine
ADL's	activities of daily living
AHD	arteriosclerotic heart disease
	autoimmune hemolytic disease
AIDS	acquired immune deficiency syndrome
a.m.	morning
AMA	against medical advice
AMI	acute myocardial infarction
amt.	amount
AP	apical pulse
ARDS	acute resp. distress syndrome
ARF	acute renal failure
	acute resp. failure
	acute rheumatic fever
ASA	acetylsalicylic acid
A.U.	each ear
BE	barium enema
b.i.d.	twice daily
BMR	basal metabolic rate
BP	blood pressure
BPH	benign prostatic hypertrophy
BPM	beats per minute
BRB	bright red blood
BRP	bathroom privileges
BSA	body surface area
BUN	blood urea nitrogen
CABG	coronary artery bypass grafting
caps	capsules

CBC	complete blood count
cc	cubic centimeter
CC	caucasian child
	chief complaint
	common cold
	creatinine clearance
	critical care/condition
CHF	congestive heart failure
cm	centimeter
CNS	central nervous system
c/o	complains of
COPD	chronic obstructive pulmonary disease
C & S	culture and sensitivity
CVA	cerebrovascular accident
	costovertebral angle
CXR	chest X-ray
d	day
/d	per day
D	dextrose
dB	decibel
D/C	discharge, discontinue
D & C	dilatation and curettage
DD	differential diagnosis
	discharge diagnosis
	dry dressing
disp	dispense
DNA	deoxyribonucleic acid
DSM-IV	Dx & Stat Manual Mental Disorders
DTR	deep tendon reflexes
EC	enteric-coated
ECT	electroconvulsive therapy
EEG	electroencephalogram
EENT	eyes, ears, nose, throat
elix.	elixir
EMG	electromyography
FUO	fever of unknown origin
g, gm, GM	gram
GI	gastrointestinal
gr	grain (about 60 milligrams)
gt.	gutta (drop)
GU	genitourinary
GYN	gynecologic

h.hr.	hour
Hct	hematocrit
HIV	human immuno virus
h.s.	at bedtime
ICP	intracranial pressure
I & D	incision and drainage
I.M.	intramuscular
IPPB	intermittent positive pressure breathing
I.V.	intravenous
KVO	keep vein open (TKO)
LLQ	left lower quadrant
LOC	level of consciousness
LSB	left subclavian
MD	manic-depressive
	medical doctor
	muscular dystrophy
MI	mental illness
	mitral insufficiency
	myocardial infarction
	myocardial ischemia
NKA	no known allergies
N.P.O.	nothing by mouth
NR	nerve root, nonreactive, no refills
	no report, no respirations
NSAID	nonsteriodal antiinflammatory drug
N/V	nausea and vomiting
OB	obstetric
OOB	out of bed
OS	oculus sinister (left eye)
OTC	over-the-counter
OU	oculus uterque (each eye)
oz.	ounce
p	pulse
p.c.	after meals
PE	physical exam, pelvic exam, pulmonary edema, pulmonary embolism
PEARL	pupils equal and reactive
per	by or through
p.m.	afternoon
P.O.	by mouth, postoperative
PP	partial pressure, peripheral pulses,

	postpartum, postprandial
	presenting problem
PROM	passive range of motion
	premature rupture membranes
pt., Pt.	patient, pint
q	every
q.d.	every day
q.h.	every hour
q.i.d.	four times daily
q.n.	every night
q.o.d.	every other day
qt.	quart
R	by rectum, respiration
RE	rectal exam, right ear
REM	rapid eye movements
R/O	rule out
ROM	range of motion, right otitis media,
	rupture of membranes
R/T	related to
RUQ	right upper quadrant
Rx	prescription
S.C., SQ	subcutaneous
Sig	write or label
SOB	shortness of breath
sol/soln.	solution
stat.	immediately
STD	sexually transmitted disease
supp.	suppository
syr.	syrup
T	temperature
TCA	tricyclic antidepressant
TIA	transient ischemic atack
t.i.d.	three times daily
TLC	total lung capacity,
	triple lumen catheter
TM	temporomandibular,
	tympanic membrane
TMJ	temporomandibular joint
UA	urinalysis
VDRL	Veneral Disease Research Lab (test)
VS	vital signs
WNL	within normal limits

ANSWERS TO STORIES

Beauty and the Ace
1. none
2. blephar
3. ante
4. dermat
5. cor
6. cut
7. cardi
8. encephal
9. crine
10. none

Joe's Adventure
1. cyan
2. dura
3. ab
4. none
5. cyst
6. none
7. antr
8. corne
9. cerebr
10. cryo
11. dynam, esthesia
12. none

The Princess in the Tower
1. bili
2. calc, crine
3. ambi, amphi
4. benign, aer
5. cervic
6. cor, eu

A Punch in Time
1. lip, or
2. part
3. lobo
4. glom
5. itis
6. osis
7. glyco
8. later
9. gram
10. none

The Great John Sullivan
1. malign
2. lal, heter
3. gran, megal
4. leio, hyper
5. lacrim
6. inter
7. gluco or glyco
8. none

Hal of "X"
1. none
2. hallux
3. lingua, megal, hyper
4. iasis, lact
5. ost
6. heter
7. inter
8. leio
9. none

All's Well with Maxwell's End
1. gen
2. maxill
3. grad
4. hormone
5. lip, leuk
6. glom, fistula, lobo
7. metabole

8. none
9. onco
10. inter

Night Fishin'

1. none
2. osmo, pachy
3. rraphy, scirr(h)
4. poster
5. phleb
6. phob, radic, pseud
7. none
8. none
9. none
10. none
11. sarco

A Gathering of Minds

1. plexus
2. platy
3. amphi
4. ment
5. histo
6. hyster
7. psycho
8. ectasis
9. lith
10. phon

The Circus

1. None
2. pre
3. phren, poly
4. thalam
5. spiro
6. trich, turbin
7. viscero
8. rrhexis
9. plast
10. none

The Case of the Latent Film

1. none
2. astr
3. none
4. ventr
5. none
6. none
7. radic
8. colpo
9. aer, fistula
10. rraphy
11. olfact, lysis
12. ophthalm or opt
13. none

A Climb to Fame

1. dynam
2. caus or caut
3. retr
4. amphi
5. pro
6. benign
7. labi
8. grad
9. ab
10. phob
11. none

The Argument

1. none
2. inter
3. trip or tripsia
4. oid
5. hyper
6. rrhaphy
7. cheil
8. phob, phren
9. aer
10. crine

The Case of the Ailing Script

1. none
2. ectomy
3. procto
4. post
5. inter
6. epi, iso
7. cine
8. cervic
9. benign
10. melan, malign
11. tympan
12. thromb, peur
13. ptosis, contra
14. none

AN INTRODUCTION TO AMBULATORY HEALTH CARE PHILOSOPHY

Stating a philosophy may predispose one to reveal his or her underlying biases, demonstrate interpretations gathered from many sources found inherently interwoven into the subject; or, in my case, represent many years of gathering information, taking histories, counseling, and working within the disciplines of orthopaedics, neuropsychiatry, and general medicine. Whatever the fundamental disciplines may have been, the philosophical metamorphosis that results must give rise to certain aspects of ambulatory health care that may otherwise go unnoticed, unheeded, or become lost forever leaving those that follow to gain their own foothold without the help of the stepping stones found and used by the many who came before. The nature of humankind is realized in the unique ability to communicate, to be a time-binding creature. Gathering together one's thoughts and casting them into the timeless sea of knowledge, hoping that these many fragmented segments of life's experience will somehow take root, grow and replenish humankind with new data to serve, save and preserve.

In support of the foregoing, I shall devote time to three modalities of thought:

1. The nursing care philosophy and self,
2. Establishing common verbal bonds with the patient, and
3. Taking a history with the patient in mind. (This will include the very specific history and total "s.o.a.p.ing" technique for a low back pain.)

Behavioral Objectives

1. Briefly discuss or identify the interpersonal or the interaction process with patients as it applies to the following:

   a. Nursing care philosophy and self
   b. Initial patient interview, obtaining an history
   c. Overall screening process, S.O.A.P.ing the patient from start to finish

163

2. Briefly describe or identify the procedure used to perform the examination of the patient with the following: Low back pain, Cold, Flu, and specific trauma to the lower and upper extremities to include at a minimum the following:

    a. Taking the history
    b. Doing the exam
    c. Deciding on an assessment
    d. Plan of action including treatment and follow-up care when necessary
    e. Final disposition

Nursing Care Philosophy and Self

Over the years, I have often asked students to take time from their studies to put together, in 500 words of less, their personal philosophy of life. For many it was a first time for this kind of thought. For some this assignment produced a startling realization that a philosophy per se, did not exist, that life was just spent against the cool winds of time. For others, it catalyzed a process already begun. For all, it gave temporary meaning to one of the moments of time, and provided direction for new thought and action, a reference point in their hierarchy of being. Nevertheless, the assignment made, they would bring them to me, the apologetic, the blushing, the dogmatic, the God fearing, the not so God fearing, the early, and the late. I read them all. Some spoke of courage. Many gave clue to a vision of the future, an insight about tomorrow seen today. They spoke of young men and women needing strength to fight their common foes, disease, ignorance, and misunderstanding. Each seemed to be aware of life and the need for love. Finally, much mention was made about the art of understanding through language and education. They all thought. They all gave something of themselves.

As you might imagine, their words in 500 or less, did not solve all the ills of our world, and they were unable to come up with any magic cures for the common maladies that inflict humankind. Instead, each in their own way, young minds, began a journey into the chilling questions of "why," and for one single moment each was given a look at "self," and having made this internal journey, they would never again be the same. Still they would go on.

A few would leave this place, their inner self-found to be in conflict with the outside reality. Others would go on to finish (in those days a forty week course), while one or two would become truly self-actualized. As instructors, we would come to know a great deal about each one who passed this way. You see, they would leave a great deal of their self behind. In this process of being here we each would come to know much about their individual philosophies. We, as instructors, would be able to see with some clarity the workings of the inner self as it struggled against the backdrop of nursing. The environment would bring out what was hidden from view. The course would bring out what was unknown. A working agreement with both must develop early if one is to stay in the flow of things. It is at this point that many began to revise their internal philosophies about life and living, and about dying. They are the ones that were able to achieve their end, graduation. What was it that they found out that kept them in the course for forty weeks?

If you expect an answer to the foregoing question that will enable you to achieve graduation without work, dream on. I suspect that students had their individual story to relate. Ones of tears, sweat, and blood. Stories that may tell of wrongs and bleached rights, of fare and foul play. Each student would have his say of the instructors. All would have their say about the course. What would make this all worthwhile is the fact that after forty weeks with this school, this faculty, there would be a change in each that would be noticed. Perhaps an inner glow would give its self away, or a certain body carriage, but always, deep within there would be a knowledge of self that was not there before, and a devotion to nursing that would only be seen as time would allow as each graduate traveled the path of life into the future and through the tangled vines of living. Each one reflecting some of what had gone on HERE. Each one taking their place in the flow of nursing. Finally, each one becoming only what they could become with such a past, fully actualized, fully alive, caring for humankind with love in their heart. This concept is better described in the following creed. It is a statement of what I feel many must come to feel if they are to be self actualized, fully involved, a valid part of nursing and life.

My Personal Creed
(A Mantra for Living)

Give me courage enough to embrace a vision of the future, keeping my mind elastic to change, always seeking to learn, then using my knowledge to aid in the healing of the sick and mending of the hurt.

Give me strength enough to stand fast against the eroding force of time, to keep myself healthy, strong and able to move against my pathognomonic foe, disease.

Give me life enough to finish what I have started, so that I shall not short change anyone in need, and that I may have time to do the best that I can, in search of man and his meaning, here and beyond this mortal vessel.

Give me love enough that I may make peace with my God, as I conceive Him to be, learn to forgive man, but never forget from where I came or where I shall finally go. I am man, transcending the beast, out of woman, a creature with speech, one who has risen above all animal expectations. Though I shall challenge Nature on all fronts, as man, I must be humble in the shadow of my creator, for in the end I shall be held accountable for my deeds done while living, be judged not by man, but by an higher force and leave behind a Heaven or Hell for those who follow, but in any case, I shall not continue in the form that you now behold.

Give me understanding enough that I shall be able to help those who wander bewildered in mental quandaries, give strength to those who need it in times of trial, and give faith to those who have gone astray in a world of confusing symbols created by man.

When all of these gifts have been satisfied, I shall be whole, for it is in the giving of myself that my true realization becomes born, as serving humankind is both my destination and my end.

Establishing Common Verbal Bonds

1. *Teaching*: Part of what you will be doing is to teach the patient since the medical jargon is usually not well known by the laity. This is to be done in such a way that you do not insult your patient, or in any way be condescending. Health teaching can be a very rewarding experience.

2. *Identifying*: You will have to identify the patient's value system in order to relate to him/her. His feedback will give clue to his background, education, and emotional state of the moment. Give him/her his/her say, don't crowd him/her with questions, make value judgements about his/her grammer or way of speaking, interrupt him/her as he/she speaks, that is, allow him/her to finish what he/she is saying. You will understand better, and he/she will feel better. You may identify something very special about each patient if you allow him/her the freedom of expression without causing him/her to guard, or in someway to splint his thoughts with things he feels YOU want to hear. Remember, it isn't YOU that is sitting there with an illness or complaint. If his/her value system is too foreign or seems incongruous to you, ask for help.

3. *Describing*: You will be called upon to describe the complaint in terms that can be understood by the patient. Remember, that you do so with the permission of the P.A., or doctor only if you are aware of their philosophy in treating patients. You will have to understand how much each patient needs to know and if you are allowed to tell it. Be clear on this. For to tell the patient something that he/she cannot handle at the time, may cause

irrevocable mental anxiety, or even create an obstinate neurosis. To designate one as a psychosomatic is for the diagnostically destitute. Remember also, that in order to describe you must KNOW and know the actual, not the supposed. Do not tell your patient stories. If you do not know, find out. If you tell a patient that you are going to do a certain thing, then please do it. This is called follow-through.

4. *Accepting*: You should accept the patient as a person without making moral or value judgements about his/her: station in life, cause of illness, or any shade of difference that may separate him/her from you as you believe yourself to be. If you cannot do this, then you should allow yourself an out. Perhaps an out from nursing.

5. *Loving*: In its broadest sense, and within the limits of your beliefs or philosophy, you should demonstrate that you care; that you care about what happens, what should be done now, and of the outcome, if within your control. Your actions, speech, and demeanor should demonstrate this. For those of you who find it difficult to "pretend," at least make an honest effort to "do." Perhaps in doing you will begin to care, and in caring you will begin to glow with what the patient will feel is genuine concern. For those of you that cannot feign even a modicum of care, or actually give a damn, then you may like mechanics better.

If the above five steps are incorporated into your clinical acumen they will have a positive effect on you patient-nurse relationship that will go a long way into the process of getting the patient well before any treatment is given: for it has been known for a long time that patients begin to feel better as soon as they enter into the treatment arena. Why not capitalize on this placebo effect, and create an atmosphere in which this feeling can flourish. Your rewards will be many, and your patient's return visits will be fewer in number and frequency.

Taking a History (Chief Complaint) with the Patient In Mind

1. *Do Not Argue*: This is no time to argue with patients about their belief, cause of illness, reason of accident, or whatever. You may wish to teach again later, or do health teaching if they have a problem that represents lack of care or knowledge about their body, health, or condition. But please do not be harsh in your manner or critical in your way of helping. You are not their stern parent figure, but instead, a compassionate human being that happens to be in the health care profession, and by all other standards, no better than they are.

2. *Own Words*: When taking a history from a patient, use his/her own words with any necessary clarification of word meaning or choice. Use quotation marks to set off their thoughts, descriptions, and phrases.

3. *Use Format*: If possible, follow some kind of format or outline until you learn the necessary steps and questions. Example: Algorithms, forms, especially the ones within this article on low back pain. These have been designed to aid you, to save time, and to assist with an assessment.

4. *Be Attentive*: Listen to your patient. Do not be so rude as to write, without making eye contact, talk to someone else, or discuss another patient on your present patient's time. If you find it difficult to remember what a patient tells you, take short notes on a separate pad and then transfer these to the form later, or during a pause. This means that you must maintain eye contact with your patient as much as is possible. If you are interrupted by a peer, ask if urgent, if not, tell him/her that you will be available as soon as you are through. Give your patient his/her due time. But remember, there will be times when a patient will want more than his/her share of your time. It will be your job to find a way to terminate the interview without making the patient feel slighted or cheated. When you can put out your hand to a patient, and they will take it, then you will know that you have earned yourself a place in the treating environment worth keeping. But, when a patient tells you "thank you" as well, you have reached a threshold in your clinical acumen that you can call self actualized, at least for the moment. There are many moments in the day of a nurse.

5. *Taber's Cyclopedic Medical Dictionary* has an interpreter index in five languages that may aid you in asking questions for those who do not speak english well; but also, this book will help you with the various meanings of many medical words.

Low Back Pain as an Isolated Entity

I. Introduction

A. *Opening Statement*: (Fable about Man's Stature) or: When man chose to stand erect, to stand on his hind legs and work against the ever constant pull of gravity with his quadrupedal motor skeletal equipment, he fell heir to the frequent inadequacies of that equipment, presupposing him to low back pain. While it is true that he has gained two hands, it is also true that he has now only two feet to do the work of four. The penalty will forever reside within the confines of his aching lower back. Let us look into some of the consequences of poor body mechanics, selective overloading, and the much talked about trauma of every day living.

B. *Objectives*:

1. Identify and/or briefly describe three causes of chronic low back pain.

2. Briefly describe and/or identify the procedure used for the taking of a history (chief complaint), performing the examination, the making of an assessment (provisional diagnosis), and the plan of action for a patient with the chief complaint of low back pain.

C. *Procedure and Lesson tie-in* (if used for class presentation):

This instruction is given in preparation for the following hours on physical assessment and examination during the screening process. The steps in the low back exam will be done and will be used as an example to demonstrate the entire procedure of taking a history (chief complaint), doing an exam, forming an impression (assessment and/or diagnosis), and discerning a valid treatment, or deciding to refer the patient to a specialist for final disposition.

II. Explanation:

A. Causes of low back pain (chronic and acute)[*]

1. Low back pain of postural origin:

   a. Poor body mechanics may account for the largest portion seen.
   b. Selective overloading of the anti gravity skeletal muscle system. The strain you can produce by over working one muscle group, especially using a cold muscle or one group because of poor mechanical advantage.
   c. Poor muscle tone or disuse atrophy. As in, because of improper use or disuse of the vastus medialis, injury to the knee occurs as it is difficult to fully extend the leg to its only stable position.
   d. Overweight.

---

[*] Ref.: Trauma, McLaughlin, W.B. Saunders & Co., 1960, Chapter 21.

2. Myositis and Fibrositis:

    a. An inflammation caused from disease or old or recent trauma.
    b. This process exists within muscle and connective tissue. It may be superficial or deep causing pain at a distance from the origin. Many times pinching massage will bring it out.

3. Osteoarthritis:

    a. If called a disease, it is one that occurs usually after forty years of age. It may be caused by an unknown factor, or be the result of past trauma, whether a gradual insult over time, or one sudden one within a few hours.
    b. It is a process of the normal aging of the adult.
    c. Usually centers its pain producing problems within the joints of the extremities. When this is so, it may be called by a special name. Reference: Arthritis. Tenosynovitis. Etc.

4. Unstable Lumbosacral Spine:

    a. Congenital defects.
    b. Transitional presacral vertebra (L-5,S-1). A most common anomaly, exhibits structural characteristics of both a last lumbar and a first sacral segment. It can be fused or have a joint interposed between the transverse process of the presacral vertebra and sacrum.
    c. Disc disease and/or trauma, as in HNP.

B. Taking a history for low back pain complaint (example):

    1. Sample History: 25 y/o cau male with hx of low back pain last 24 hours. States that he has had no injury within the last five years. Patient remembers helping to lift heavy tent the day before the episode. However, he denies pain at the time of lifting. Pain began the following morning after getting out of bed. Pain is made worse by standing and lifting things. Pain seems to respond to heat and being flat on back. Patient's daily habits and job: works at a desk all day, does very little exercise during the week. Plays some handball and used to lift weights. pain is located low back and does not radiate into either leg. Has been seen for a similar type pain over five years ago. Was not hospitalized. Does not remember if he was given any medication at that time. Was told to exercise, but does not remember how. Is not taking any medication at present. Patient appears to be in good health and walks with a list to the left. Patient is 6'0" weighing 200 pounds. No other complaints.

Any family history of bone disease may well fit in at this point. Be sure to watch the patient's affect, posture, and listen to the words that he uses to describe his malady.

C. Physical Exam (objective data) patient with CC low back pain:

1. Use chronological record of care form.
2. Guide to Physical Exam

a. *Spine Alignment*: Objective signs of LBP are loss of normal lumbar loridosis called *flattening*, or a lateral list causing asymmetry of the lorodotic line.

b. *Muscle Spasm* defining the erector spinae muscles palpable as prominent hard cord in a position of maximum stretch. Some my say that there is no spasm in the back. Describe what you feel and can see.

c. *Mobility of trunk*: (ROM) Loss of motion in the quadrupedal position, usually in the lorodotic region. Loss of ROM in flexion and/or extension with some associated pelvic tilt. Using a plumb bob one my calculate how much pelvic tilt or shortening of the lower extremity exists.

d. *Deep Tendon Reflexes* (DTRs): Biceps, C-5 level; Triceps, C-6 level; Radial, C-8 level; Ulnar, T-1 level; Patellar, L-2 & 3 level; and the achilles, L-5-S1 level.

e. *ROM Exercises*: SLR, straight leg raising; WLR, weight load resistance; Sit-ups with legs straight and also with hip flexed; Heel-toe walking to test for strength of the muscles supplied by the nerves mentioned in (d), and to define any existing paresis or imbalance.

f. *Sensation*: "Normal" feeling within each lower extremity. This is a subjective data since you will have to ask the patient.

g. *Atrophy*: Check one muscle group against the opposite side, usually the thigh group or the calf group are chosen. Measure an equal distance from a known body landmark, mark with pen, and use a tape measure to determine the girth of the muscle mass. Palpation of some muscles during use may give clue as well.

h. *Sciatic Pain*: Attachment of the hamstring muscles to the pelvis flexes the lumbosacral joint and stretches the paravertebral soft tissue putting tension on the sciatic nerve. Certain motions of the hamstring muscles will bring out pain in a tender inflamed sciatic nerve. If the nerve has been traumatized, it will also be tender. Direct pressure with a blunt instrument or digit may bring pain along the sciatic distribution as well. During straight leg raising dorsiflexion of the foot may bring out sciatic pain, and if so, this should be noted. Sciatic pain, whatever the method used to elicit, must be evaluated.

D. Forming an Impression (Dx or Assessment):

1. After taking an accurate history and doing a rather complete exam, which should take about 15 minutes, an assessment, or provisional diagnosis, will naturally follow. Some low back complaints will take longer than 15 minutes. If there has been an history of recent injury or the patient has been seen by someone the day before you will have to make some changes in your format. If the patient is in pain from an injury, you may want to defer part of your exam. In the absence of obvious disability, a referral to a specialist may be indicated. At that point it is necessary not to create further trauma.
2. The assessment should be based on ruling out specific entities, especially neurological and/or traumatic findings. In the presence of any positive findings, a specialist or doctor should make the final disposition.
3. The following assessments are made most often:

    a. Lumbosacral strain.
    b. Lumbosacral strain with muscle spasm.
    c. Lumbosacral pain, etiology unknown.
    d. Low back pain of postural origin.
    e. Low back pain (chronic or acute) post traumatic.
    f. Rule out disc disease.

E. Treating the Isolated Entity:

1. In the absence of any positive neurological signs, and with a negative history for trauma, treatment will be primarily symptomatic with concern directed to obviate the cause, reeducation of the involved muscles, rest, exercises, and the medication of choice.
2. Isolation of the offending muscle group may be possible in some cases. When this feat is accomplished the treatment may be exacting. The treatments listed below are by no means the only ones, for even as I put these words on paper, new ones are being tried somewhere.

    a. Ice massage alone, or on an intermittent basis with heat.
    b. Rest on a firm, thin, mattress, supine or laterally recumbent. Not on abdomen.
    c. Pelvic traction.
    d. William's exercises.

    e.   Pain medication with muscle relaxant, non narcotic.

    f.   Dichlorotetrafluroethane or ethyl chloride topographically. Surface anesthesia, similar to ice massage technique.

    g.   Injection of a trigger-point with xylocaine and depo-medrol or some other kind of anti inflammatory medication.

    h.   Patient teaching.

III. Summary:

A. Review of Main Points:

    1.   Causes of low back pain.
    2.   Taking a history for low back pain as a chief complaint.
    3.   Objective exam.
    4.   Forming an assessment.
    5.   Treating the isolated entity.

B. Closing Statement:

When low back pain is the chief offending complaint, certain observations will point the way to probable cause, and possible treatment. Knowing the possible causes, using a thorough history, and doing the exam should create an environment for positive treatment in all but the most resistant cases. A specialist or an orthopaedic doctor sees lower back syndromes existing outside these confines. A specialist in neurology or orthopaedics will inevitably make final judgment in all equivocal cases. Your job is to see that this determination is made before the offending lesion produces irreversible damage to the patient.

In this paper I have given clue to the complexities within the treating arena that exist as soon as the patient enters the room. Your job is made complex in no small way because you can speak, think, and form pre judgments in more than just the area concerned with your patient's signs and symptoms; but, equally because you are human and subject to the same feelings, wants, and fears as your patient. Objectivity, though often sought by many clinicians, may not be the answer. Many a machine can give an impression. Emotional involvement does not mean that the loss of effectiveness must follow. Too much of our world today is given to the superficial, "I do not want to become involved," type of verbal, and body communication. We have become cold diagnostic computers aloof, alas, even oblivious to our human surroundings. If one seeks no one, no one need respond. Each patient is part of your life whether you want him or her to be or not. Treat that person as an end in his or her self, for every one has some value of merit. We are all part of a whole. If you take from that whole, you take from yourself. The reality of living is that we are born needing someone and we will certainly die quite alone without someone to care. Many will come to a clinic for no other reason than needing someone to care, even if for only that moment. The fruits of healing are deeply interwoven with the care given to the mind as well as the body, and the body and soul are one.

EXAMPLE OF LESSON PLAN
PSYCHIATRY

I. Introduction:

    A. Read Schizophrenic Places

    B. Today, Mental health is going down. The foregoing poem is part of series of poems written as "California Mental Health is Going Down." This can be found in the learning center. Please check it out and read it if you get a chance.

II. Explanation:

    A. Show the DSM-IV

    B. Relate a little about each:

        1. Psychiatrist (4 years med school) and then a varying number of years learning their craft.

        2. Psychoanalyst (3 to 5 years learning techniques in the process of psychoanalysis.

        3. Psychologist (minimum of a master's degree) in one of several specialties.

    C. Tests to Evaluate Mental Health:

        1. Wechsler Adult Intelligence Scale

        2. Stanford-Binet Intelligence Scale

        3. Thematic Apperception Test (TAT) also, tell a tale. This technique is known as a projective test. Another example is the Rorschach test.

    D. Clinical Symptoms:

1.	Amnesia	9.	Dysphoria
2.	Anxiety	10.	Euphoria
3.	Apathy	11.	Hallucination

4. Autism   12. Labile
5. Compulsion   13. Mania
6. Conversion   14. Mutism
7. Delusion   15. Obsession
8. Dissociation   16. Paranoia

E. Freudian Interpretation of a reality thought to be.

1. Id, a representation of unconscious instincts and psychic energy present at birth and represents the child.
2. Ego, mediates between the demands of the id and the realities of the external world. (Compare with adult and self) The ego is the central control or decider system of the personality and is said to operate in terms of the reality principle.
3. Superego, the outgrowth of learning the taboos and moral values of society. In essence, the superego is what we refer to as the conscience, and is concerned with good, bad, right, and wrong. (Compare with parent)

The primary weaknesses in many of Freud's axiomatic conclusions about man may have been his lack of scientific method. Many of his case studies were based on but one person, a process that leads him to much introspection. But, some say that from such a great intellect, a little introspection may reveal much. I am not so sure.

TREK THERAPY

BY

William J. Russell

Wouldn't it be great if just watching a TV program gave you the equivalent of one hour of therapy, and this therapy has provided you with an aftermath of well being? Made you feel better each time you watched the program. Well, that may not be too far from actuality.

In the 1960s there was a personality theory called transactional analysis. Developed initially by a psychiatrist, Eric Berne (1961, 1964), and popularized by Thomas Harris (1969) a psychiatrist. Transactional analysis is essentially a procedure for evaluating interactions between people regarding three ego states: child, adult, and parent. An individual is seen as having potentials in all three of these ego states, but in any particular situation with another person, he may be found usually in one of those states. Thus, John may be a child in relationship to his wife, dealing with her symbolically as though she was his mother; and, with his friends, he may be a parent taking a supervisory role. If we look at only the implication that these three ego states represent; the parent, one who cares and is in charge; the adult, one who is logical, and often sees things as black and white; and the child, who is playful, and can be quite illogical at times, we can see endless combinations as the three states interact.

On the other hand, what if we can observe these three states interacting before us in the form of a play, movie, or TV program? And what if this TV program is Star Trek? Consider the three ego states as individuals. James Kirk represents our parent figure. Mr. Spock plays the adult, and the Child is Dr. "Bones" McCoy. In each episode, these three characters interact while solving some problem of space, time, or state of being. As we watch these three personalities interact, we find our self-drawn in to the situation at hand. As the play comes to a climax, we too feel the situation, by identification. Finally, when all has been solved, completed, and the end is before us, we feel whole. In the process of watching we have drawn these three parts of our own self together. And for the moment, we are whole. We feel good, at least, until we get another fix with the next episode.

III.   Disorders:

A. Anxiety Disorders
B. Delirium and Dementia
C. Dissociative Disorders
D. Eating Disorders
E. Mood Disorders

1. Bipolar I and II
2. Cyclothymic
3. Dysthymia
4. Major Depression

F. Personality Disorders

1. Antisocial
2. Borderline
3. Histrionic
4. Narcissistic
5. Paranoid
6. Schizoid

G. Schizophrenia (possible handout)

H. Sexual and Gender Identity Disorders

    1. Exhibitionism
    2. Fetishism
    3. Pedophilia
    4. Sexual Masochism
    5. Sexual Sadism
    6. Transvestic Fetishism
    7. Voyeurism

I. Somatoform Disorders

    1. Hypochondriasis
    2. Conversion Disorder

IV.   Therapeutic Intervention

A. Psychotherapy

    1. Behavior therapy
    2. Family therapy
    3. Group therapy
    4. Hypnosis
    5. Psychoanalysis
    6. Sex therapy

B. Electroconvulsive Therapy (ECT)

    1. Especially for major depression with suicidal ideation that is uncontrolled.

C. Drug therapy

    1. Antianxiety and antipanic agents

        a. benzodiazepines
        b. selective serotonin reuptake inhibitors (SSRIs)

    2. Antidepressants
    3. Antipsychotics (neuroleptics)

        a. phenothiazines

4. Hypnotics
5. Mood stabilizers (lithium)
6. Stimulants

V. Closing Statement:

The primary mental illnesses that exist within our society, ones that cause the most disturbing byproduct, are mostly the ones regarding psychotic behavior; namely, schizophrenia & bipolar illnesses. While the others are also important, it would be a great relief if we could find the cause for schizophrenia. Probably a better word would be schizophrenias. The plurality of the word reveals to us that the disease is not just one syndrome, but many. Perhaps finding just that one would also reveal many others. We can only hope.

CONTRIBUTIONS

Back when this course was 17 weeks long I would allow the students to write a story of their own using the mnemonic devices and association/images found in the book. I would jokingly tell them that it was their chance for immortality. Of course, these stories would be for bonus point, 10 points for each story. They were allowed a maximum of three. This would give them a possible 30 bonus points. It was a good practice then, and would still be today. With this course going through the stages of change, from 17 weeks, to a distant learning course that would only have five meetings and finally becoming an online course, it seems that this procedure may be lost. The following named students have had their work used in this book by their permission and because their work was outstanding.

Bojorques, Kathy, *Joe's Adventure*, 1994
Cook, Lynde C., *All's Well With Maxwell's End*, 1997
Hall, Isabel, *The Circus*, 1994
Newbury, Deborah, *The Great John Sullivan & Night Fishin'*, 1999
Taylor, Shirley, *The Princess In The Tower*, 1998

BIBLIOGRAPHY

Chabner, Davi-Ellen. "The Language of Medicine." W.B. Saunders Company. 2004, 7th edition.

Dorland's Illustrated Medical Dictionary. W.B. Saunders Company. 1981, 26th edition.

Ehrilch, Ann. "Medical Terminology for the Health Professionals." Delmar Publishers. 1997, 3rd edition.

Glazier, Teresa Ferster. "The Least You Should Know about Vocabulary Building Word Roots." Holt, Rhinehart & Winston, Inc. 1990, 3rd edition.

Harned, J.E. "Medical Terminology Made Easy." Physician's Record Company. 1968, 2nd edition.

Skinner, Henry Alan. "The Origin of Medical Terms." The Williams & Wilkins Company. 1949, 1st edition.

Tabers Cyclopedic Medical Dictionary. F.A. Davis Company. 2001, 19th edition.